Style Eyes

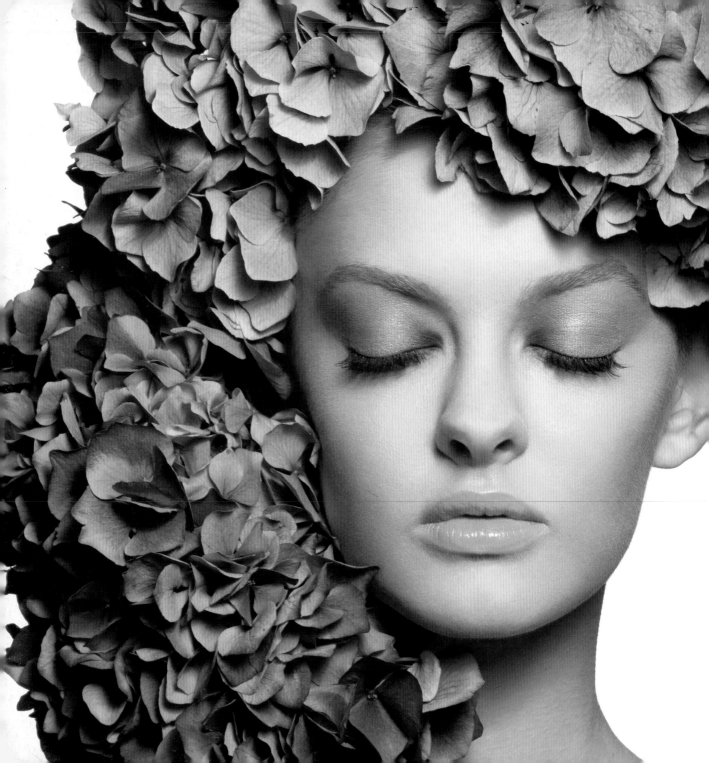

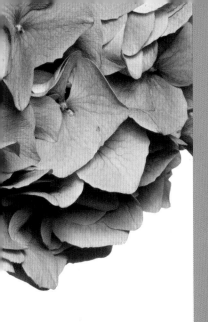

Style Eyes

Taylor Chang-Babaian

Beauty Photography by Albert Sanchez
Creative Direction by Pedro Zalba

A PERIGEE BOOK

A PERIGEE BOOK
Published by the Penguin Group
Penguin Group (USA) Inc.
375 Hudson Street, New York, New York 10014, USA
Penguin Group (Canada), 90 Eglinton Avenue East, Suite 700, Toronto, Ontario M4P 2Y3, Canada
(a division of Pearson Penguin Canada Inc.)
Penguin Books Ltd., 80 Strand, London WC2R 0RL, England
Penguin Group Ireland, 25 St. Stephen's Green, Dublin 2, Ireland (a division of Penguin Books Ltd.)
Penguin Group (Australia), 250 Camberwell Road, Camberwell, Victoria 3124, Australia
(a division of Pearson Australia Group Pty. Ltd.)
Penguin Books India Pvt. Ltd., 11 Community Centre, Panchsheel Park, New Delhi—110 017, India
Penguin Group (NZ), 67 Apollo Drive, Rosedale, North Shore 0632, New Zealand
(a division of Pearson New Zealand Ltd.)
Penguin Books (South Africa) (Pty.) Ltd., 24 Sturdee Avenue, Rosebank, Johannesburg 2196, South Africa

Penguin Books Ltd., Registered Offices: 80 Strand, London WC2R 0RL, England

While the author has made every effort to provide accurate telephone numbers and Internet addresses at the time of publication, neither the publisher nor the author assumes any responsibility for errors or for changes that occur after publication. Further, the publisher does not have any control over and does not assume any responsibility for author or third-party websites or their content.

First edition: August 2010

Library of Congress Cataloging-in-Publication Data

Chang-Babaian, Taylor
  Style eyes / Taylor Chang-Babaian ; beauty photography by Albert Sanchez ; creative direction by Pedro Zalba.
    p.   cm.
  "A Perigee book."
  ISBN 978-0-399-53596-3
  1. Beauty, Personal. 2. Eye—Care and hygiene. 3. Cosmetics. I. Title.
  RA 778.C3764 2010
  646.7'26—dc22   2010015393

PRINTED IN THE UNITED STATES OF AMERICA

10 9 8 7 6 5 4 3 2 1

Neither the publisher nor the author is engaged in rendering professional advice or services to the individual reader. The ideas, procedures, and suggestions contained in this book are not intended as a substitute for consulting with your physician. All matters regarding your health require medical supervision. Neither the author nor the publisher shall be liable or responsible for any loss or damage allegedly arising from any information or suggestion in this book.

Most Perigee books are available at special quantity discounts for bulk purchases for sales promotions, premiums, fund-raising, or educational use. Special books, or book excerpts, can also be created to fit specific needs. For details, write: Special Markets, Penguin Group (USA) Inc., 375 Hudson Street, New York, New York 10014.

To my family, who are always there for me.

To the women I meet, who continue to teach me with their beautiful faces and inspire me to grow.

And to all the other people who support me, without whom none of this would be possible.

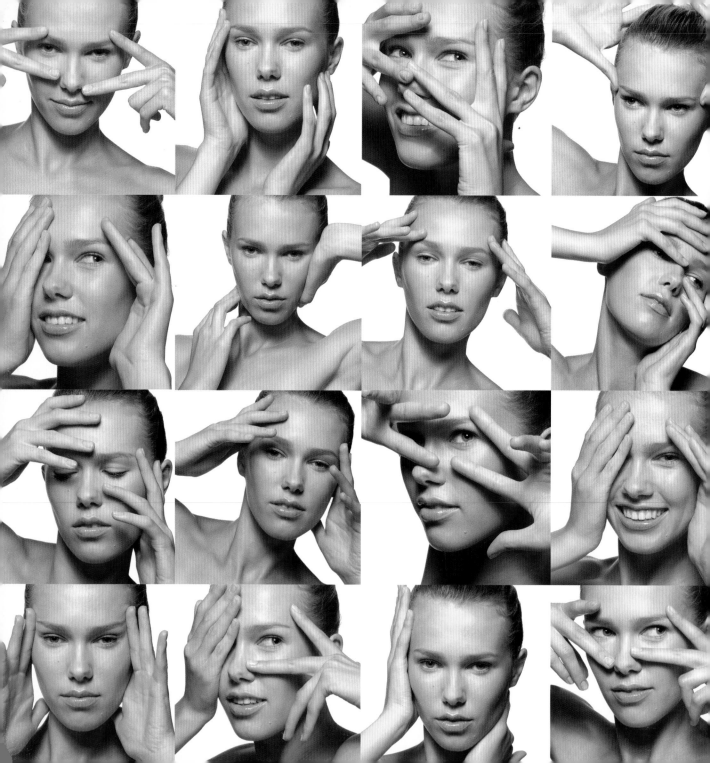

Contents

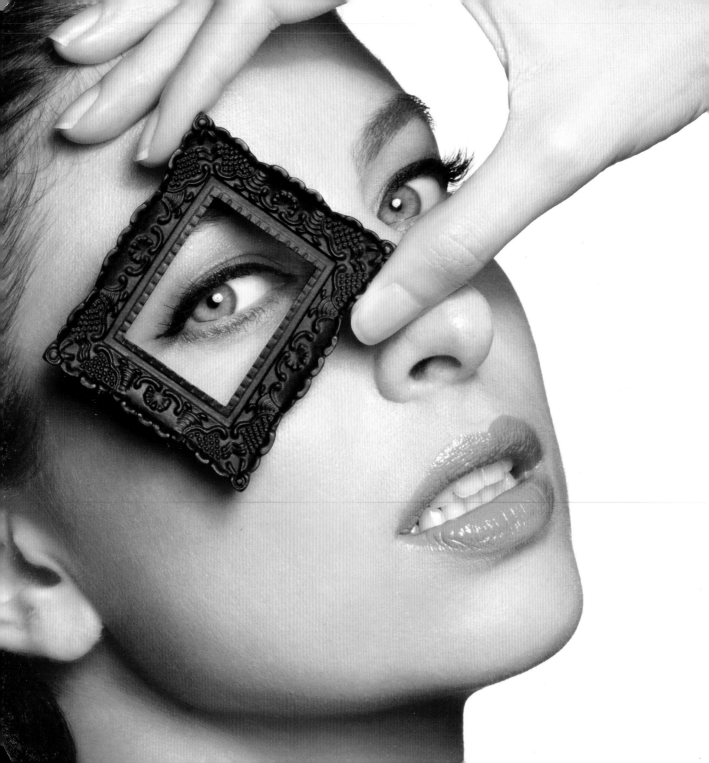

Introduction

The eyes are the windows to the soul. It's a cliché, but it's true. What is your soul saying? More often than not, it's saying, "I'm tired and I could really use some concealer!" Applying eye makeup can be a nerve-racking experience, but also an incredibly rewarding one. While traveling throughout the country talking to thousands of women, I've learned that the confidence level when it comes to eye makeup is overwhelmingly low.

That's why I've created *Style Eyes*. A quick swipe of eyeliner in the right direction can take years off your face. Another quick swipe of concealer can give you the appearance of a full night's sleep. I've been told countless times, "Wow, it's like magic!" Nice sentiment; however, I am no magician. I am a makeup artist, and being an Asian woman with small eyes, I've spent decades playing with eyeshadows and liners, mascaras and primers. After much trial and error, I've come to discover that eye makeup is really quite easy once the various tools and techniques are broken down and explained, as I have done for you. Whatever your beauty concern—small or deep-set eyes, dark shadows, monolids, thin or full eyebrows—I've included easy tips and tricks to help you create beautiful eyes and eyebrows, no matter what your age, skin tone, eye color, or eye shape is. You'll find it fun and empowering to experiment with new looks and techniques—and if you don't like something, simply wash it off.

This is no ordinary makeup guide. Not just full of pretty pictures, this book will help you understand the composition of the eye and eyebrow, teach you why you should choose one specific shade over another based on the look you are trying to achieve and the color and shape of your eyes and eyebrows, and offer simple step-by-step instructions to achieve professional-quality looks for all ages and occasions. Even if you think you've mastered your current eye makeup look, there's always more to learn and new techniques and products to explore. Eye shapes change; age, lack of sleep, or even the wrong meal can change the shape of the lid, creating puffiness and sagging. You'll learn tips and tricks to fix these challenges and more, simplify even a smoky eye (a classic but sometimes tricky-seeming technique), and add new color to your repertoire.

You may feel that you know the basics of eye makeup and decide to skip straight to the amazing looks featured throughout. But if you're still a novice, or if you find yourself with questions, it's best to read the earlier chapters to understand the basic techniques utilized. And in the end, do what's comfortable for you. If you've never worn eye makeup (and I've met plenty of you out there), try something natural. Even just a hint of makeup—perhaps some well-applied mascara under a perfectly groomed brow—can make a world of difference. Once you're comfortable with an everyday look, take some risks and experiment. And remember, if you don't like it, it's only makeup. A cotton ball and about thirty seconds are all you need to start over and try again.

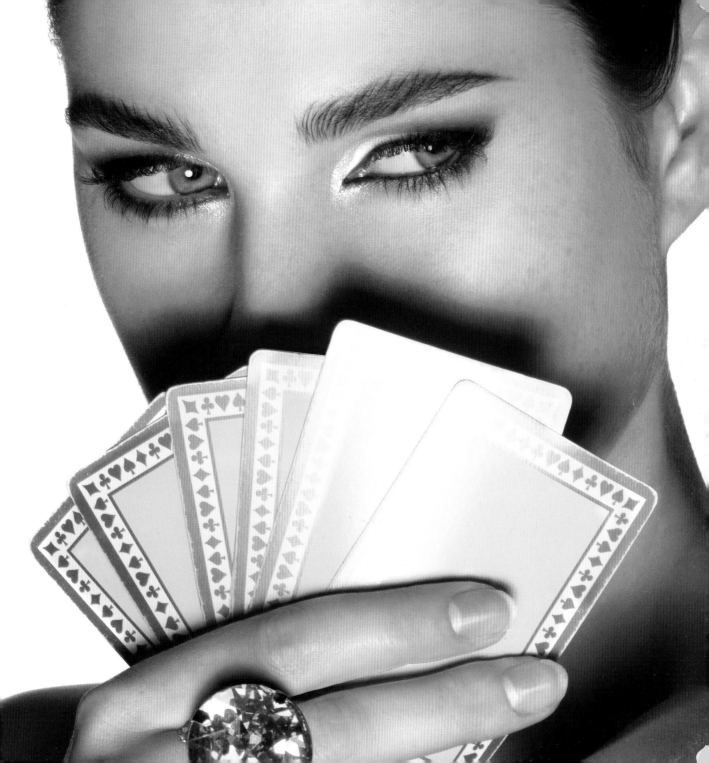

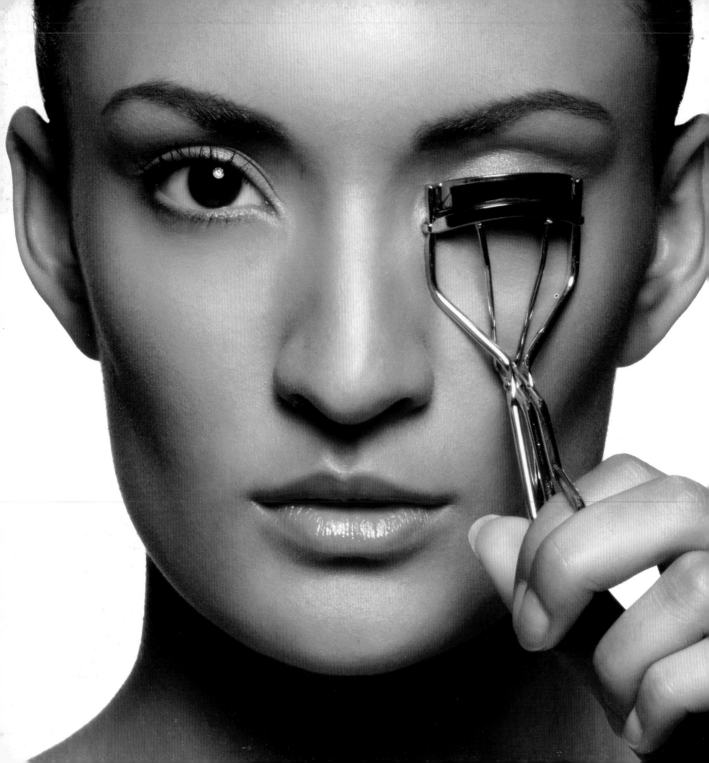

Beauty School: Proper Eye Care

Eye and Skin Care

Caring for Damaged Skin

Before starting any great eye makeup application, examine and prep the skin. This ensures that you'll get the smoothest application possible and minimize imperfections in the skin, such as fine lines or spots.

The skin around the eyes is incredibly thin—a fraction of the thickness of the rest of your skin. This is why signs of aging show first around the eyes as fine lines or crow's feet. It's important to treat the area from the brows to the cheekbone delicately (something to think about the next time you rub your eyes or decide to skip the eye cream).

Sun Damage

The sun is a big contributor to most eye area problems. Darkness, fine lines, and milia (see page 3) all get worse with sun exposure. To minimize the effects of the sun, make sure to always use sunscreen. One designed for the eye area is best. During summer months or on especially bright days, wear sunglasses that block both UVA and UVB radiation for added protection of both the skin around the eyes and the retina. During prolonged periods of sun exposure, such as long walks, gardening, or days out on the beach, add a hat to your ensemble.

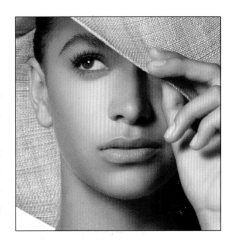

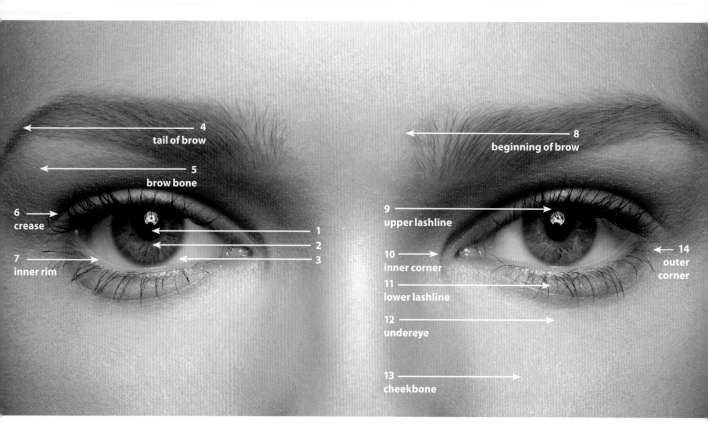

4 tail of brow
5 brow bone
6 crease
7 inner rim
1
2
3
8 beginning of brow
9 upper lashline
10 inner corner
11 lower lashline
12 undereye
13 cheekbone
14 outer corner

EYE STRUCTURE

1. Pupil—the dark part of the eye. Minimizes with light and increases in darkness.

2. Iris—the colored part of the eye. The color can change.

3. Sclera—the white part of the eye.

4. Tail of the brow.

5. Underside of the brow bone—the top of the orbital bone.

6. Crease—the natural indent of the skin, sometimes referred to as the eyelid fold.

7. Inner rim—the inside line of the eyelid, between the eye and the lashline.

8. Beginning of the brow.

9. Upper lashline.

10. Inner corner of the eye, closest to the nose.

11. Lower lashline.

12. Undereye—the thin skin area under the eye, inside the orbital bone.

13. Cheekbone.

14. Outer corner of the eye, closest to the temple.

Milia

Milia are the white bumps that are most often found directly under the eyes. They are caused by several factors, including heredity, eye creams and makeup removers that are too thick or heavy for your skin, and sun exposure. Dead skin cells get caught in pores and trapped by a layer of skin, creating the characteristic appearance. To minimize and prevent milia, be sure to exfoliate the skin under the eyes using creams and eye masks that contain gentle acids, retinols, and/or vitamin C; use sunscreen, eye creams, or serums that are light in texture; and avoid thick creams that are not meant for the eye area or that contain pore-clogging ingredients such as mineral oil.

Fine Lines

When we're young, our skin renews itself naturally, as cells turn over quickly. But as we get older, the cell turnover slows, and dead skin cells build up around the eyes. The skin thins and collagen breaks down, reducing the elasticity in the skin and causing lines. Fine lines can be minimized by using eye creams and eye masks that promote cell turnover and help rebuild collagen. Our cells regenerate while we sleep, so it's essential to apply eye creams in the evenings.

Oily Eyelids

Women with oily lids tend not to get as many fine lines or wrinkles. But it is more difficult for them to wear eye makeup, as the oiliness causes cosmetics to smudge or crease. Waterproof mascaras and eyeliners will minimize any smudging. Dust a layer of silica-based powder on the lids before applying eyeshadow to absorb excess oil. Stick concealers tend to take longer to melt, so use a small amount of concealer instead of foundation to prime lids for makeup. If the mascara on your upper lashes tends to smear on your lower lids, try curling your eyelashes (see page 29).

Taylor's Tip

Avoid splashing your eyes with very cold or very hot water or rubbing your eyes when you're tired—either of these actions can increase fine lines and break capillaries. Try a pressure point massage instead. This has been a part of Eastern medicine for centuries and is a great way to improve circulation in the eye area. Using your middle finger, gently apply pressure to the pressure point areas around your orbital bone and hold each pressure point for three to five seconds. These points are located at the middle of the brow bone, on the upper and lower temples, at the middle of the top of the cheekbone, and along the sides of the nose near the inner corners of your eyes. Begin above the brows and repeat as necessary.

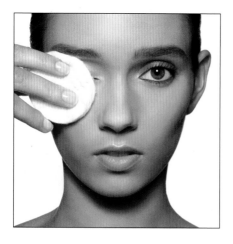

Take It Off: Essential Eye Makeup Removal

When dealing with layers of primer, concealer, eyeshadow, eyeliner, and mascara, using a gentle and effective eye makeup remover is vital. Look for oil-free removers that are made specifically for the eye area. If you wear waterproof eye makeup, make sure your eye makeup remover also works on waterproof mascara. Apply remover to a cotton pad and swipe gently over closed eyelids beginning from the inner corner to the outer corner of the eye. Repeat as necessary using clean cotton pads. Use cotton swabs for the hard-to-reach areas, such as under the eyes, along the lashline, and the inner corners. You can also use pads that are presoaked in remover. They can be a little messy, so remove excess solution with cotton pads. Tissues can be too rough for the delicate eye area, so stick with softer cleaning tools, such as cotton pads and cotton swabs.

Preventing Eye Infections

The eyes are sensitive and prone to infection. A few simple precautions will help guard against uncomfortable, unsightly, or potentially serious complications:

- Always use only cosmetic and skin-care products that are designed specifically for the eye area.
- Avoid touching your eyes with your hands whenever possible. If you have to touch your eyes, make sure to wash your hands and nails thoroughly first.
- Wash your hands often in general. Because our hands touch everything, it's important to keep them clean not only for our eye health but also for our overall body health.
- Keep all of your cosmetics clean, and replace caps whenever they are not being used.

- Don't share cosmetics with other people, especially mascaras and eyeliners.
- Don't sleep with eye makeup on. Remove any bits of makeup using eye makeup remover and a cotton pad, then close your eyes and wash the eye area with a gentle cleanser and rinse thoroughly.

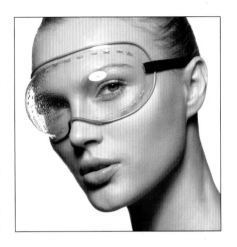

Makeup Counter Cleanliness

The store makeup counter can house tons of bacteria, putting you at risk for many viral and bacterial infections, including sties and conjunctivitis. The ideal way to test colors and textures is on the back of your hand whenever possible. However, if you must try something on, take these precautions to greatly reduce the likelihood of infection:

- Don't double-dip disposable mascara wands. Mascaras are most likely to cause infection, as they stay wet and bacteria can grow in the tubes. You're better off buying mascara and trying it at home—just make sure you know what the return policy is.

- Sharpen all eye pencils to remove any remnants of used eyeliner from the previous use. If a sharpener is not displayed on the makeup unit, be sure to ask for one. For twist pencils, break off the tip if possible or roll on clean tissues until several of the outer layers have been removed.

- To test eyeshadow, use a cotton swab or disposable sponge to wipe off the grimy top layer from the display tester. Then follow with a second disposable sponge to test the eyeshadow itself.

- To test a brush, request a clean one and wipe it on a clean tissue to ensure it hasn't been used. Make sure brushes are clean if someone is helping you with the application. Don't be shy about asking; it's important to your eye health.

- Scrape off the top layer from concealer tubes with a makeup scraper and discard. Apply a small amount to the back of your clean hand to work with, instead of allowing the tester to touch your skin directly.

Veins

Visible veins in the eyes can be caused by irritation from cosmetics, environmental factors such smog or allergens, or a lack of sleep. To reduce the appearance of veined or bloodshot eyes, follow these steps:

- If you've slept with your eye makeup on, remove all makeup, cleanse, and rinse thoroughly. If possible, allow your eyes to rest and don't use makeup for a day or so.

- Use eye drops. They come in a variety of strengths, from simple washes such as saline, allergy, and redness formulas, to the strongest ones, which contain menthol. Eye drops contain ingredients that quickly constrict capillaries and make eyes look whiter instantly. Check the label and make sure that the product is FDA approved. Read all the directions carefully, and avoid sharing bottles with others.

- If you have a foreign object, such as an eyelash or a dust particle, in your eye, close the eye and allow it to tear. It's a great way to flush out the eye naturally.

- If redness lasts longer than a few days, see a doctor; changes in the eyes can be a sign of other things happening in the body.

- Stay away from pink and purple eyeshadows. They will intensify the redness in the eyes.

Sensitive Eyes

Most often, sensitive eyes are not sensitive at all; rather, poor makeup hygiene is to blame.

- Throw out mascara after two months.
- Use disposable mascara wands to avoid contaminating the tube.
- Don't double-dip into cream or gel eyeshadow jars.
- Use plastic makeup scrapers or the back of a clean brush to pick up any products that are in a pot.
- Sharpen eye pencils before each use to remove any remnants of contaminants from the previous use.
- When using twist eyeliners, roll the eyeliner on clean tissue paper several times to remove the outer layer before and after each use.
- Talk to your ophthalmologist to see if you have a specific allergy.
- Don't apply moisturizers too close to the eye. The skin will absorb eye creams and moisturizers into a larger surface area than originally applied, so they may bleed into the eyes if applied too close.
- Avoid glitter and flakey mascaras that can fall into the eyes and irritate them further.
- Avoid hard eyeliner; all liners should glide on gently. Hard eyeliner is probably made of an inexpensive wax that is not good for the eyes. Splurge a little for products around the eye area.
- If you tend to get a lot of shadow in your eye, try a cream-to-powder eyeshadow.
- Look for hypoallergenic makeup, which is ophthalmologist tested for sensitive eyes.
- If your eyes tend to tear, use waterproof gel eyeliners and mascaras. They don't move, so they will not smudge into the eyes.

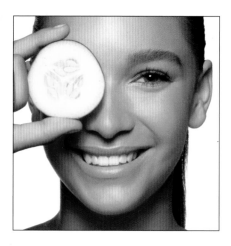

Puffy Eyes

The appearance of puffiness is most often due to the swelling of tissues around the eyes. It is often caused by:

Too much sleep (or not enough sleep)

Fluid retention

Excess salt intake

Pregnancy, which often causes edema

Alcohol and tobacco consumption

Thyroid disease

There is another type of puffiness, which is caused by loose skin and excess fat, not swollen tissue. The collagen breakdown of the layer of tissue that holds the fat in the eye weakens and also causes drooping and sagging.

To temporarily reduce puffiness caused by swollen tissue:

- Drink plenty of water; this will flush out excess salt and toxins, such as alcohol and tobacco.

- Cut out tobacco completely; not only is it better for your body, but your eyes will look much younger.

- Cool compresses constrict blood vessels and prevent the flow of fluid into the tissues. Teas such as chamomile contain natural anti-inflammatories that reduce swelling. Place two used teabags in the refrigerator until cool. Place teabags on closed lids for fifteen minutes.

- Sliced cucumbers are also a good cool compress, as they contain natural tannins that reduce puffiness. Take out clean, cold cucumbers from the refrigerator, cut into half-inch slices, and place on closed eyelids for ten to twenty minutes.

- Get your rest; try sleeping on more than one pillow to keep your head elevated during sleep. Make sure to sleep on your back, not your stomach, so fluid doesn't flow into your face.

Taylor's Tip

Avoid cold water or cold compresses. Anything too cold can pop capillaries around the delicate eye area.

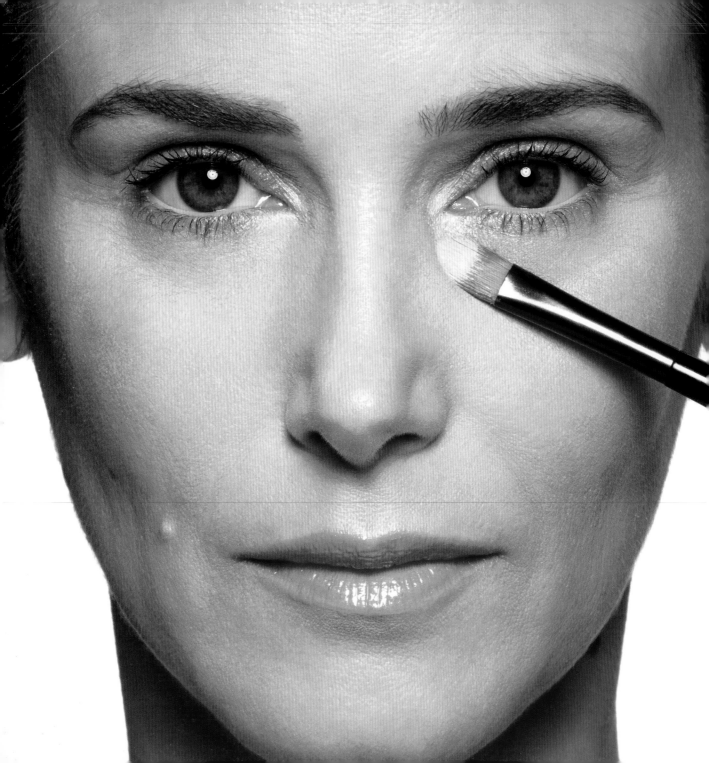

A Clean Slate: Preparing the Canvas

Taking the time to apply the appropriate foundation to the eye area not only makes the eyes look better but can actually make makeup last longer. A few extra minutes spent in the morning can extend your great eye-makeup application by several hours.

The Perfect Concealer

The perfect concealer can change the eyes completely by evening out skin tone and texture and brightening the eyes, giving the illusion of livelier, youthful eyes.

Often when applying concealer, women make the mistake of thinking that dark circles under the eyes should be covered with the lightest concealer color possible, which can result in a light grayish halo on the skin under the eyes. Instead of using concealer several shades lighter than your natural skin tone, look for a concealer only a half shade or at most two shades lighter than the skin color directly beneath your eyes. If you have very dark undereye circles, look for a concealer a shade or two lighter than the color of the skin on your cheekbone directly underneath your pupil.

Then look at the color of your undereye circles. If the imperfection is pink or red in color, choose a concealer with a yellow undertone. The

Taylor's Tip

Apply foundation first on lids and undereyes, then apply concealer where necessary. This minimizes the amount of concealer application. Using as little of the heavier concealer product as possible creates a more natural look. For mature skin, use a thinner, creamier concealer. This minimizes wrinkles and darkness without looking cakey. Avoid applying too much powder under the eye, as this will define lines.

yellow will cancel out the redness. If it's brown or black, choose one with a pink undertone; if it's blue, choose one with slight orange undertones.

Dark skin often needs concealer with more orange or slightly red undertones, as darkness will generally appear as deeper shades of the natural skin tone, making pink an ineffective concealer color. Look for the lightest color on your face and find a heavy cream concealer one-half to two shades lighter. For very pale skin, use concealers that have a slight yellow undertone, as skin can be thin and have a pink or purple hue under the inner corner of the eye.

To identify what undertone a concealer has, try laying out several swabs of different concealers side by side. The differences in undertones will appear more obvious when next to each other. Or simply try one on in the store and see if it is doing the job—if not, you need a different concealer.

Concealers should be applied with your fingers or a small concealer brush (I prefer synthetic short brushes made of high-quality taklon) for precise coverage. Brushes are easier to get into the hard-to-reach areas of the eyes, such as the inner corners—especially if you have deep-set eyes. However, the natural heat of the fingers softens the concealer, making it easier to blend.

Types of Concealers

Cake

Cake concealer is very dense in texture and opaque in coverage. It can be used to cover very dark circles and even bruised eyes. However, it can look heavy, so using a light touch is essential. Avoid setting with a lot of powder, as it can look thick and unnatural.

Stick

This concealer has a similar texture to a cake concealer but is less dense, and it provides medium to heavy coverage. Higher-end stick concealers are moisturizing and yet dry enough that applying additional powder

The search for the right concealer never ends. As skin textures change due to weather and age, different concealers can be necessary throughout the year. Balance out skin texture by looking for wet or cream concealers for dry skin. Skin gets drier with age and often during winter months. Stick concealers are great for oily skin as well as hot and humid weather during summer months.

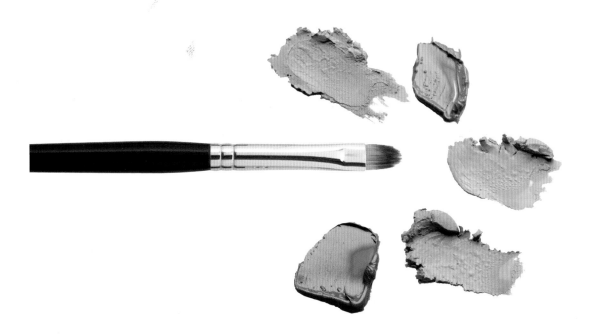

isn't necessary. This is my choice if the weather is warm, or if you have a problem with concealers rubbing off. Because it has a high level of pigment, a little goes a long way.

Pen

These concealers are very light in texture but can cover light to medium dark circles. They're usually the best for fine lines under the eye or on thin skin because they don't build up and make the skin look crepey.

Cream

I like this creamy, butter-like texture better for the undereye area, as it contains more moisture than a cake concealer and is more pigmented, which is great for concealing dark circles. It provides medium to heavy coverage and comes in a tube or pot. Heavy cream concealer is also effective on dark skin.

Taylor's Tip

When choosing a concealer, keep this in mind: The lightest concealer is pen, followed by cream, stick, and finally cake, which is the heaviest concealer.

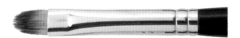

Concealer Brushes

Large

Use large concealer brushes for the undereye and inner corners of the eyes closest to the nose, as well as the eyelid area when concealing visible veins. Look for sable or synthetic brushes that are flat and rounded at the tips to fit into the contour of the eye. Soft tapered edges make for easier blending. Use with concealer like an eraser to clean up fallen eyeshadow.

Small

Small concealer brushes are useful for targeting a more precise area, such as the small dark-spotted areas under the inner corners of the eyes. These are also great to use with a tiny bit of concealer as an eraser to clean up eyeliner mistakes on the outer corners of the eyes.

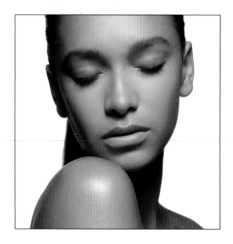

Hiding Dark Circles

It's not just lack of sleep that causes dark circles. I recall going to a photo shoot and working with a young Hollywood celebrity who was known for his edgy look, characterized by dark undereye circles. I started to wonder if he was really just that overworked and underrested. While contemplating this, I met his beautiful three-year-old daughter, who had the same dark circles. Clearly it is hereditary in that family. Quite often thin skin, which results in visible blood vessels, or excessive melanin (skin pigment) production in that area is the cause of dark circles. But whether your undereye "bags" are hereditary or a result of your lifestyle or environment, these simple tips can help reduce them:

- **Exercise** will increase circulation and pump oxygen into the vessels, which will help blood flow. This is important, as often dark circles are caused by not enough oxygen getting to the veins.

- **Vitamins**, particularly iron supplements, can be effective. Often iron deficiencies will cause dark circles. Try liquid iron rather than pill form to help control iron loss and get more oxygen into the veins.

- **Water** will flush out toxins in your body that can cause dark circles, so be sure to drink plenty of it.

- **Eye masks** that contain vitamin C as well as vitamin K are a great way to minimize dark circles. They inhibit melanin (pigment) production for those who have dark circles owing to natural pigmentation.

- **Sunscreen-infused eye creams** are crucial to protect the undereye area from sun exposure. The sun thins out already thin skin under the eyes; sunscreen helps minimize further thinning of the skin as well as future darkness that can be caused by tanning of the undereyes.

- **Brighteners** are great for instant gratification. They have reflective properties that lighten up the eye, often containing mica to add a slight shimmer to the undereye area.

- **Sleep** is probably the most effective method of reducing dark circles. Cells heal at night, so give your eyes a break and get your eight hours.

- **Cold cucumbers** placed over the eyes are a natural astringent and shrink and constrict the body tissues.

- **Black tea** contains tannic acid and caffeine, constricting vessels to minimize any dark veins that are showing through the skin under the eyes. They may stain light or very dry skin, so moisturize before applying cold tea bags to your eyes.

- **Blush** is a great way to add life to the face. Dark circles can make you look unhealthy and tired. Blush provides a distraction from those dark circles and gives the illusion of instant health. While smiling, apply blush using a small blush brush to the apples of the cheeks under the orbital bones of the eyes. For light skin, try pale pink blush; for medium skin, try a hint of bright pink; for dark skin, use a berry shade; and for dry, dehydrated skin, use cream blush in the appropriate shade.

Taylor's Tip

For the best coverage on the undereye area, apply concealer directly to the dark region and gently blend to the edges using your finger.

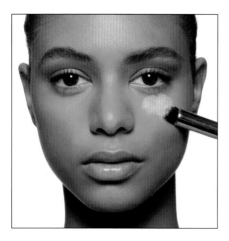

Setting the Eye Area

Setting Foundation on Eyelids

You need to use foundation on the eyelids as well as under the eyes for a couple of reasons, the main one being that it allows makeup to stay on throughout the day by priming the lids. Setting foundation means to apply powder on top of foundation so that the foundation does not move. This creates a smoother surface on which to apply eyeshadow, thus minimizing blotchiness, and keeps eyeshadow from smudging or fading throughout the day.

Choosing a Powder

When setting foundation on eyelids, apply powder gently on top of foundation before applying eyeshadow.

Loose Powder

For the eye area, use loose powder, which is lighter in texture than other powders. It sets the lids without adding thickness. Use a translucent loose powder with no color or a hint of yellow for light to medium skin tones, as powders will slightly darken when layered on top of foundation. So, be sure to choose a shade lighter than your foundation color. Women with darker skin may have to accommodate their skin tones and use a lighter powder for the undereye area, so look for powders that contain yellow or orange undertones.

Pressed Powder

Pressed powder is the best type of powder to keep with you during the day for makeup touchups because it doesn't create a mess. However, most pressed powders contain oils and binding agents to hold the powder in place, which can magnify fine lines in the eye area. To ensure a softer application, rub off any excess powder from the puff before application.

Undereye Powder

Undereye powders often have an extremely fine texture. Using a powder that is finely milled with a very soft texture under the eyes is essential if the skin under your eyes has fine lines or is dry. More and more companies have developed specific undereye powders. I prefer the translucent kind that contains a slight shimmer.

Powder Tools

Powder Puff

Puffs deposit the most powder, which can create an overly cakey look. To get a lighter application, pick up powder with the puff and rub off the excess on your other hand. To apply it under the eyes, press the puff gently onto the skin in a rocking motion (like a boat rocking over waves). Puffs are great for travel, if you have to touch up at work, or during a night out on the town.

Powder Brush

Using a brush is my favorite way to apply powder, as it gives the most controlled application and deposits a small amount of powder. When applying powder, choose a soft, high-quality powder brush. The best options are brushes with hairs made of taklon (a high-end synthetic fiber), squirrel, or sable for the delicate skin under the eyes. Avoid rough brushes; not only will their bristles irritate skin but they will not deposit powder evenly. Pick up powder using your brush, shake off any excess by lightly tapping the handle with your finger close to the bristles, and apply powder onto entire closed eye in a swiping motion, from the inner corner to the outer corner of the eye. I like to apply powder to the rest of the face first, then to the eyes, so that I get a lighter application of powder.

Cotton Swabs

If you need something quickly and all your brushes are dirty, cotton swabs are great for applying powder under the eyes, as they deposit small amounts and can get close to the eyes.

Taylor's Tip

I use small powder brushes in the undereye area to get closer to the eyes without getting powder in them. You can also use a clean eyeshadow brush.

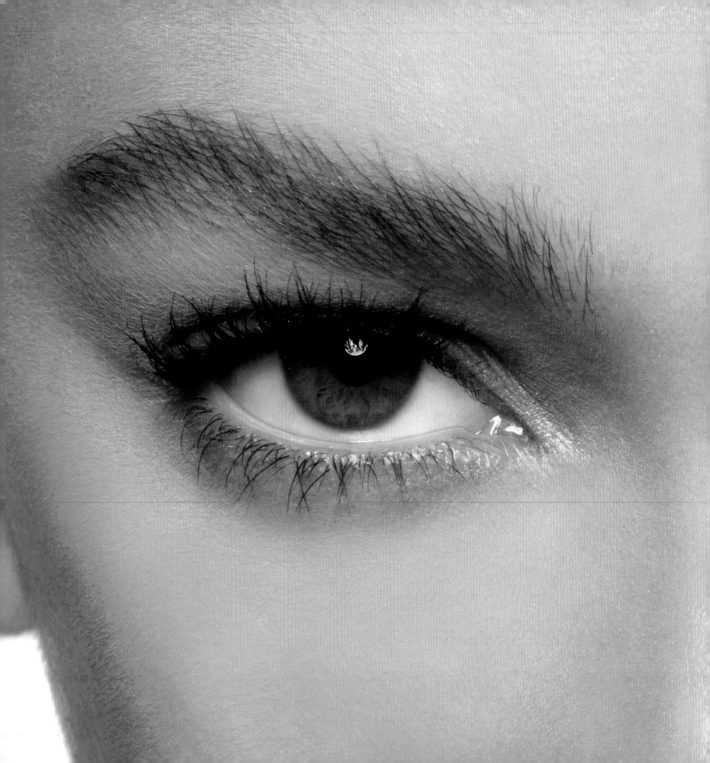

Creating the Perfect Frame: Brows

Brow Basics

Eyebrows are essential to beautiful eyes. When shaped well, they can add symmetry to not only your eyes but your entire face. They have the capability to make you look softer, polished, and even younger.

Shaping Brows

To determine the proper shape for your eyebrows, keep the following in mind:

1. Place a brush vertically along the side of your nose and slightly outside the corner of the inner eye. The brow should begin here.

2. The arch should begin above the outside of the pupil.

3. To determine where the brow should end, place a brush diagonally from the nose to the end of your eye. The brow should end at the point the brush hits.

4. For close-set eyes, start brows farther away from the bridge of the nose. (See page 21.) For wide-set eyes, start them closer to the bridge.

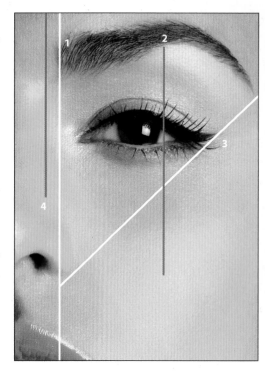

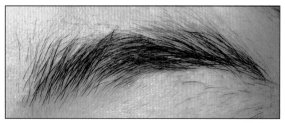

Before

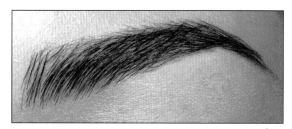

After

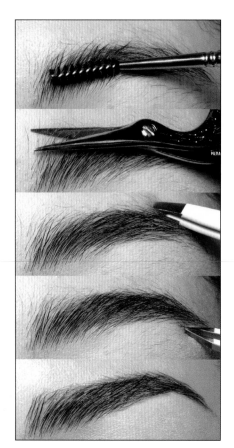

Brush brows up to smooth out brow hairs.

Cut hairs going against the growth. Look for scissors with short blades to avoid accidental overcutting. If the end of the brow grows down and refuses to go up, brush only the ends of the hairs down and carefully cut into shape. You may have to cut the ends first before tweezing some of the unwanted hairs under the arch and at the end of the brow.

Tweeze above and below the brow if necessary. Use white liner to determine the tweezing area if you are not sure where to tweeze and need a guide. Cover stray hairs with liner to see how the brow will look once they are tweezed.

Step away. Sometimes when you are staring only at the brows, you can forget to check how they frame your eyes. Check in a large mirror several times during the process to see how the brows look in relation to your entire face.

Close- and Wide-Set Eyes

If the width of your eye doesn't fit in between both of your eyes, more than likely you have close-set eyes. If your eyes are far enough apart that you can imagine fitting a third eye between them with room to spare, your eyes are wide set. Determining this is important when deciding where the brow shape should begin to create balance. For close-set eyes, start brows slightly farther apart (toward the temples) than above the inner corner of your eyes to bring the eyes farther apart. For wide-set eyes, start the brows closer to the bridge of the nose, giving the illusion of bringing the eyes closer together.

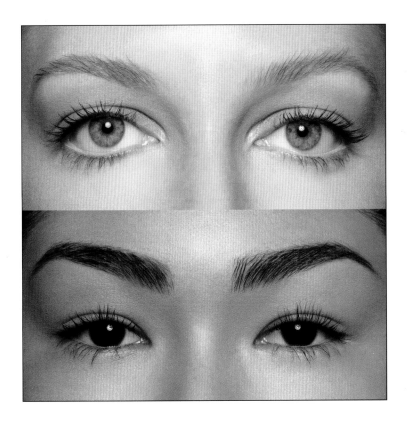

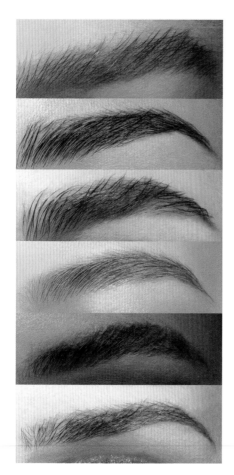

Full and Arched

Full brows are in fashion again. Keeping them brushed up gives the look a hint of edge. (See page 83.)

Strong Arch

This is probably the most popular of eyebrow looks. This brow shape gives the eyes the illusion of lift. (See page 20.)

Full and Short

Adding extra length to shorter, unruly brows can create shape, rather than tweezing and cutting length away. (See page 72.)

Delicate

Brows that are thin and delicate just need a hint of powder to create a finished look. (See page 56.)

Round

Not everyone's brow looks good perfectly arched. If you have large eyelids, try bringing the arch of the brows down a bit to create balance. (See page 53.)

Thin

If the distance between your brow and eye is fairly small, this brow is best, as it gives the illusion of a larger eyelid. (See page 74.)

Taylor's Tip

Work with what you have. If you have thin, rounded eyebrows, only arch them slightly if you want them to look natural.

Brow Hair Removal Methods

With so many different methods of removing brow hair, here's some help choosing which one is best for you.

Shaving

Brow shavers look similar to barbers' razors, but on a much smaller scale. They are great for removing lots of hairs quickly when you can't tweeze, but the hairs don't grow back fine, as they do with waxing or tweezing. Brow shavers are very sharp, so you need to be careful. Make sure to use a cream to protect the skin.

Stringing

A popular method in the East, stringing uses simple strings intricately placed to crisscross and pull out unwanted hairs. Many people swear it is less painful than tweezing. Make sure to go to a reputable salon; I've seen some less-hygienic technicians hold the string in their mouths.

Tweezing

Tweezing is my all-time favorite brow hair removal method. I'm very picky about each and every hair I pull, so tweezing gives me the luxury of taking my time and being precise. Look for high-end tweezers with tips that close completely.

Waxing

The skin around the eye area is so delicate that waxing can be a tricky method, but sometimes it's the only option, especially for brows with many stray hairs growing closer to the forehead (a common problem). As waxing removes hairs quickly, there is no room for error. A more precise method is to remove most of the area outside the eyebrows first with the wax and leave the questionable areas for tweezing.

Brow Grooming: Products and Tools

Brow Powder

This is the best product to create softer-looking brows. Use powder at the beginning of the brow to create softness and a pencil (see below) at the end of the brow for definition. Powder is best applied with an angled brow brush. Eyeshadow can also be used for this purpose, but brow powders have a different texture and pigment level, and will last longer.

Brow Cream and Pomades

Cream creates a defined brow. It is especially great for filling in very sparse areas because it's more opaque and can give the illusion of more brow hairs. For a more natural look, use the cream sparingly, as it packs a powerful punch with just a little product. It's best to apply it with a thin angled brow brush made of synthetic material.

Brow Pencil

Brow pencils generally last longer because they contain waxy ingredients that prevent the color from sweating away. They are great for creating definition at the ends of the brows. Many brow pencils have spiral brushes or dense angle brushes on the opposite side of the pencil. Use them to brush out any hard lines created by the pencil and create a softer look.

Brow Gel

Brow gel gives brows an instant finished look, especially if your eyebrows grow downward or are difficult to tame. Use the gel sparingly and don't touch your brows after they're set. Brushing the set brow gel can cause it to flake off.

Colored Brow Gel

Colored brow gel not only offers variety but also covers up gray hairs and temporarily lightens dark eyebrows, which can soften eyes dramatically. Colored brow gel is a great way to add color to seemingly lifeless, pale eyebrows. Look for a brow gel no more than two shades darker than your natural brow color for a more natural look.

Tweezers

When buying tweezers, make an investment and buy a professional brand, not just your local drugstore's version. Tweezers come in slanted, flat, and pointed shapes. The pointed style is best for those really hard-to-get hairs. The slanted style is great for everyday, all-purpose grooming, since you can angle the slant to get close to the hairs you are tweezing. Stick with the flat heads to apply false eyelashes.

Scissors

Scissors can be used for eyebrows that have a tendency to be more difficult to control or grow downward at the ends. I like small, straight scissors, preferably stainless steel. Look for types made specifically for brows, with short blades to avoid overcutting.

Brow Stencils

Brow stencils are cutouts of different eyebrow shapes that are placed over eyebrows to show where to fill in and where to tweeze. They can also be used for simple maintenance after getting brows professionally groomed.

Brow Brush

This is an essential tool used to brush up and smooth out brow hairs. This brush usually comes in the shape of a toothbrush or a spiral. I prefer the spiral shape for thinner brows and for more detailing of the brows, and the toothbrush shape to brush up full brows.

Spool Brush

The spool is a spiral-shaped brush similar to a mascara wand but with shorter, even bristles. It is a great brush for cleaning up excess mascara and smoothing out fine-to-normal brows or removing excess sculpting gel from eyebrows.

Bristle Brush

The bristle brush looks like a toothbrush and is great for grooming thicker eyebrows because it gets deeper into the brows, straightening out even the deepest layers.

Small-Angle Brow Brush

Look for short, semistiff bristles to fill in brows with powder. I also like synthetic bristles when working with creams or to create a sharper angle.

Choosing a Brow Color

When choosing a brow color, consider your natural brow color and add a hint of your hair color to your eyebrows for a uniform look. For example, if you have blond hair and brown eyebrows, look for a color that's in between to create flow from your face to your hair.

Brows that are too dark can make you look harsh, creating a frowning effect. When applying brow products, fill in any holes in the brow first—because the initial touch of powder or pomade to your brows deposits the most color, it's necessary that that initial deposit be where any holes in the brows are, then the excess can be used at the beginning of the brow.

Easy Brow Fixes

Hook Eyebrow

The "hook" eyebrow is one where the arch begins too close to the beginning of the brow, and it is a common error. After seeing them in several states and on even the most fashionable women, I finally asked a dear friend, who simply said she thought the arch was supposed to start where her eye began. Fortunately for her and many like her, the hook eyebrow is also one of the easiest to fix. Simply connect the beginning of the brow to the peak of the arch and fill in. If the eyebrow is too full, tweeze under the beginning of the brow, then connect and fill in.

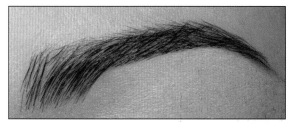

Before

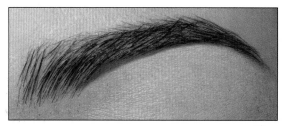

After

Thin Eyebrow

Overplucking is another common trend and can look unnatural. It often creates a dated look and reminds me personally of eyebrows in the 1930s. To correct this common problem, until brows grow in I like to use an eyebrow pencil or pomade and apply it in short strokes, duplicating the look of brow hairs. Avoid overdrawing brows, as this can look fake. Fill in only where necessary.

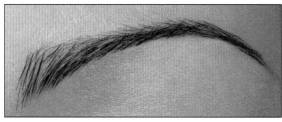

Before

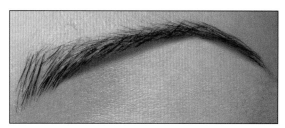

After

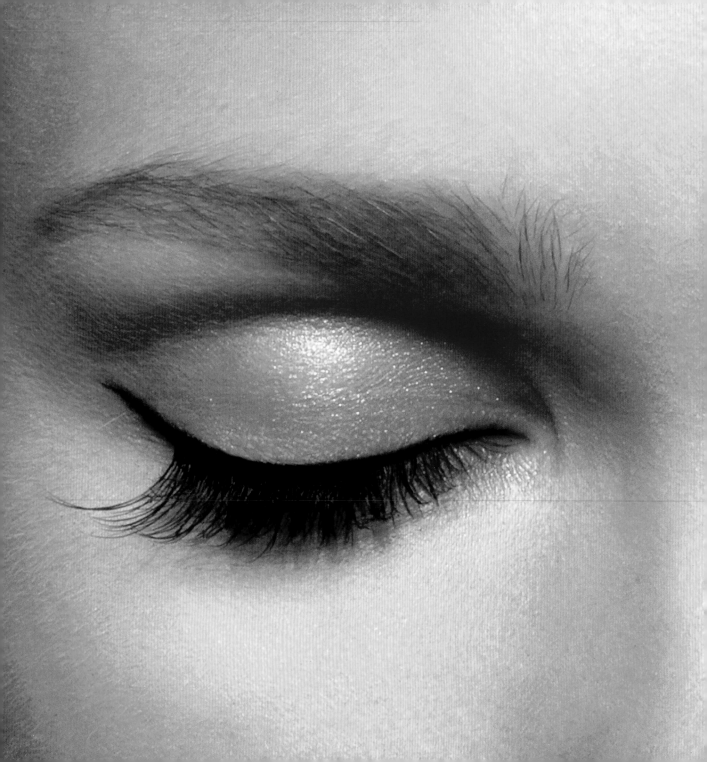

Line Up, Lash Out: Lashes and Liners

The Pro's Guide to Eyelashes

Eyelashes are the final step to beauty. They add youthfulness and femininity to any great makeup look. Whether you're looking to lengthen, curl, or add thickness, these steps will help you bat your lashes with confidence.

How to Curl Your Lashes

1. To get the best results, make sure that your eyelashes are clean and free of any old mascara.

2. Open the lash curler and place the entire upper lashes into the curler while looking down into a mirror. Slowly close the curler as near to the lashline as possible without pinching the skin. After making sure the curler is holding all the lashes, squeeze gently (squeezing tightly will cause lashes to crimp) and hold for five seconds. Most eyelashes will curl in just a few seconds.

3. Open the curler and move it halfway up the lashes. Squeeze it closed gently for an additional two to three seconds.

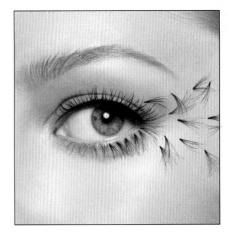

Taylor's Tip

You get what you pay for when it comes to lash curlers. The best results are obtained with high-end metal lash curlers, such as those found in department stores.

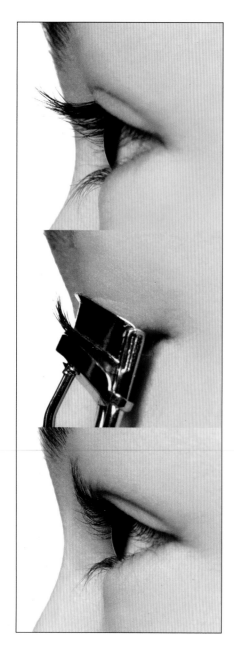

4. Open the curler for the last time and move it close to the tips of the lashes. Curl for another second. Doing this makes lashes curl into a C shape, duplicating naturally curly lashes. Curling only at the base of the lashes can result in an L shape, which doesn't look as natural.

5. Follow with mascara. (See below.) After mascara, your lashes should not fall; if they do, your mascara is too heavy for your lashes. Try a waterproof formula, which helps lashes retain the curl.

The Right Mascara for Your Lashes

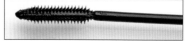 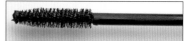

Fine or Sparse Eyelashes

Mascara wands that have close-set bristles will add volume to sparse lashes. Mascara that is too heavy will make fine eyelashes fall. Look for brushes with short, wide-set bristles and product that doesn't appear to be dripping wet. For lashes that can handle a bit of weight, try using mascaras that contain fibers to add volume and length. Look for mascaras with ingredients such as nylon. You can usually see fiber-like materials on the wand. If the first coat is not weighing the lashes down and seems to be doing its job, feel free to apply another coat for additional volume.

Falling Lashes

Waterproof mascara is the best option for lashes that tend not to hold a curl, as it is often lighter weight than standard mascaras. Use a silicone-based eye makeup remover specifically made to remove waterproof mascara.

Taylor's Tip

Use eyeliner along the lashline to give the illusion of fuller lashes. Set with dark shadow for a longer-lasting look.

Full Eyelashes

Very thick eyelashes can sometimes overpower the rest of the face when mascara is applied. Look for tinting mascara. Thin and short silicone bristles (most mascaras will show the bristles on the package) are also great for lengthening lashes without adding fullness. Look for key words such as "natural" or "lengthening." Wipe off the wand carefully before applying to remove excess mascara for a thinner, more even application.

Long Eyelashes

On lashes that don't require any extra length, look for long bristles that are farther apart, with key words such as "separating" on the package.

Choose the mascara wand that will provide the type of application you need:

- Wands that have bristles that flare out in several directions will add volume.
- Wands that have thin spiral bristles get to hard-to-reach areas.
- Wands with straight bristles will separate lashes.
- Combs deposit color well, but aren't as good for volume.

Wear waterproof mascara on the lower lashes if your mascara has a tendency to smudge.

Mascara Application

1. While looking down into a mirror, apply mascara starting at the base of the lash and gently wiggle to push the bristles into the lashes, and follow through to the tips of the lashes.

2. Allow the first coat to dry completely, then apply a second coat. Try applying to the outer corners of the lashes only, to make eyes appear more lifted.

Taylor's Tip

There are now thousands of mascaras to choose from. Fortunately, most mascaras will state on the package or in their advertising the properties of the mascara and the brushes. Pay special attention to key words on packages.

Taylor's Tip

If your lashes fall into multiple categories (for instance, they are both short and fine), try applying two different coats of mascara (in this case, start with lengthening mascara and then add volumizing).

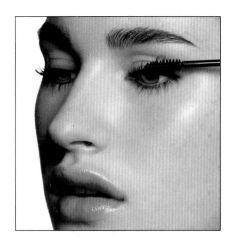

Advanced Lash-Enhancing Techniques

Lash Extensions

Lash extensions are expensive and high maintenance, but they may be worth the cost for people who don't wear eye makeup daily and have the money and time for upkeep. Real hairs are affixed to existing hairs using special glue (they have to be attached to natural hairs, so this might not be worthwhile for people with sparse natural lashes). This must be done by a professional who has been specifically trained to do lash extensions. The extensions can be attached to both the upper and lower lashes. Lash extensions can look so natural that it's difficult to see where the real lashes begin and extensions end. Extensions take a few hours to apply and last one to two months; touch-ups also have to be done in between, usually after two weeks, for any hairs that may have fallen off. It's even better, however, to get them touched up weekly; without regular touch-ups, the hairs twist around and can't be pulled off manually. Great care is necessary when working with lash extensions: Do not use makeup that contains any form of oil, cream shadows, some liners, and mascara; be very careful when applying liner and shadow; and never rub your eyes.

Eyelash Tinting

Tinting should be done at a reputable salon, as it can cause blindness if performed incorrectly. Mostly applied using vegetable dyes, tinting darkens lashes but doesn't add bulk. Women with paler lashes can consider this as an alternative or in addition to mascara, as it makes such a dramatic difference with or without makeup. Lash tinting should be done every month and is relatively inexpensive. If you have blond or pale lashes, you just might love it!

Eyelash Perming

Think of this as similar to a regular hair perm. Lashes are wrapped around small rods to curl them up. Personally, I notice very little difference in results between this and an eyelash curler—in fact, I think a quality metal eyelash curler works a thousand times better. Call me old school, but I prefer mascara and a curler. Another drawback to eyelash perming is uneven growth. Lashes fall out continually, and new eyelashes usually appear every two months, so straight lashes could appear alongside permed ones, requiring constant maintenance.

Special Lash Growers

The latest in eyelash technology, these prescription treatments were developed after doctors treating glaucoma patients discovered that one of the side effects of the glaucoma drops were longer, thicker eyelashes. They took the main ingredient, bimatroprost, and created a cosmetic product that's packaged similarly to liquid eyeliner and is applied every evening onto the lashline. These products are very expensive, with a tube running about $140 for a month's supply. The results are significantly better when applied consistently. While there are nonprescription lash growers on the market, the prescription ones do work better. You will have to go to your doctor to get a prescription, and make sure any lash growers you use are FDA approved. It's important to read the instructions very carefully and be aware of side effects—in particular, people with light-colored eyes may see their eyes permanently darken. The skin close to the lashline can also darken.

False Eyelashes

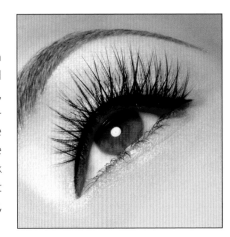

I absolutely love false eyelashes and don't think they get the attention they deserve. They add femininity and sexiness to any eye and are used on most fashion photo shoots, runways, and red carpets. In the sixties, false eyelashes were a staple of the makeup routine. Sadly, later generations have lost the knack for them. Women are often afraid that false eyelashes will make them look retro and ridiculous. But today's false lashes are almost undetectable from real lashes and can make eyes look more alert and larger, all while looking natural. With so many different types of false lashes on the market, it's easy to achieve any desired look, from everyday to glamorous and dramatic.

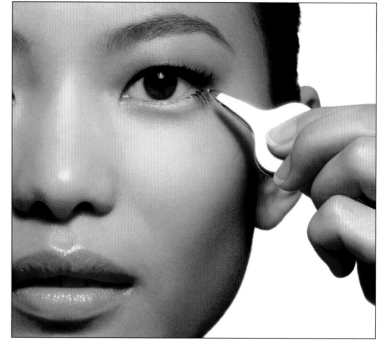

Taylor's Tip

When cutting false lash strips to size them to your lid, sometimes you don't know which end to cut. I prefer to cut the outer corners to make the most natural look.

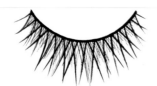

False Lash Strips

Some women find lash strips too fake-looking, and in the past that may have been true, as false eyelashes were often modeled after retro looks. However, eyelash strips have evolved and can look completely natural and very versatile. They come in dozens of different styles. Some offer a retro look; others crisscross at the base, duplicating the look of natural lashes, and are almost undetectable. It's now hard to tell where natural lashes end and false ones begin. When looking for strips, pay attention to the shape of your eye. Women with wide-set eyes should look for lashes that are longer in the middle of the strip and taper at both ends. This will open up the eyes instead of further widening them. If eyes are more close set, choose lashes that are shorter in the middle and longer at the ends of the lashes. This draws eyes out. When in doubt, try a few different styles to see what works best.

Lower Lashes

Lower lashes are great for strong period looks, such as the 1960s look, and can also be worn for a night out on the town, but always with a smoky eye and upper lashes as well so that they look more natural. If you have sparse lower lashes, lay the strip on top of your existing lashes; otherwise, apply it beneath your lower lashes. You can also use individual eyelashes that are shorter than upper individual eyelashes.

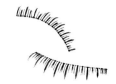

Individual Lashes

Individual lashes are clusters of hairs attached together at one point that flare to create the most natural look and are great for women who want very light enhancement to their lashes. Sometimes all a woman needs is three or four individual lashes on the outer corners to "wing out" the eye or a few in the center to add height and open up the eye. Women with very sparse lashes should stick with strip lashes as they will hold longer and are easier to apply on a sparse lid.

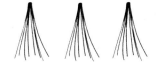

Single Lashes

These are individual hairs—just one, or sometimes two—that are applied to the lashline. Use these for a truly separated lash look, but note that they are more difficult to apply and do fall easily into the eyes, as they don't have natural hairs to sit on. Use a strong eyelash glue to keep them attached.

Three-Quarter Strip Lashes

These types of strip lashes are a favorite of mine because they fit almost every eye and are very comfortable to wear (no poking, as sometimes happens with full lash strips). They are easier to apply than full strips, as they don't need to be cut.

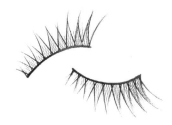

Corner Lashes

These lashes were designed to add just a little lift to the ends of the eyes and create a dramatic look, extending and accentuating the outer corners. They are a great way to add a little oomph to your lashes without using a complete strip. Apply as you would an eyelash strip.

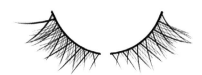

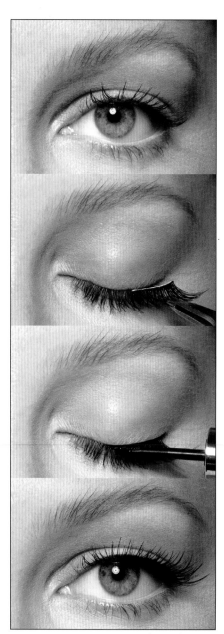

Corner Lash Application

Lash Glue

Be careful in choosing the correct lash glue. The glue should not be too runny or too strong—glue that is too strong can make the lashes very painful to take off, which is terrible for the delicate eyelid area. Very strong glues tend to be clear and have noticeable fumes when opened. A better option is glue in a tube that comes out white or iridescent and dries clear.

How to Apply False Lash Strips

Applying strips correctly can take time and practice. I like to apply false eyelashes *after* all of my eye makeup has been applied. This should be the last step, as applying makeup on top of false lashes can cause them to lift off.

1. Gently curl eyelashes if necessary (if you have straight or semistraight eyelashes).

2. Apply mascara. (Curling lashes and applying mascara give the lashes something to lie on, so you won't have to hold them in place.)

3. Apply glue along the base of the strip. Allow the glue a few seconds to get tacky.

4. Balance the strip on top of the eyelashes, attaching false lashes as close to the lashline as possible. (If necessary, use the back of your tweezers to push lashes closer to the base.) Cut eyelash strips in thirds to allow for easier application. This allows you to apply them in a connect-the-dot fashion. This is a great solution for those who have a difficult time balancing entire strips on their lashes. Apply on the lashline beginning at the inner corner of the eye, and connect from the inner corner to the outer corner. If the last strip is too long, cut accordingly.

5. Allow to dry for fifteen seconds and open the eye gently, making sure that glue has not stuck to the lower lashes. If it has, use a wet

pointed cotton swab and run between upper and lower lashes to remove the glue.

6. Once the glue has dried clear, apply a liquid liner to smooth out the upper lashline and cover any remaining glue mark or sheen. Alternatively, curl your lashes after you have already applied the false lashes. This will allow the fake and existing lashes to blend together, making them also feel more comfortable. With both techniques, use black or brown liquid eyeliner if necessary to darken the glue line after the glue has dried.

7. If you make a mistake, simply remove the false lashes, remove the excess glue from the false lashes, and reapply. Remove any glue remaining on your lid. If it doesn't all come off, no worries. It will dry clear and be nearly undetectable.

Eyeliner

Eyeliner is one of the harder cosmetics to apply and can take some practice, but the rewards are worth it. Eyeliner can make the most dramatic difference in the shape and look of an eye. Eyeliner options used to be slim. Liquid liners were too runny, and pencils were hard and painful to work with. The way I kept eyeliner on when I was younger was to burn an eyeliner pencil and wait for it to cool slightly before applying it. More than once I was in a hurry and burned myself. Luckily, such dangerous practices are no longer necessary. Today's eyeliners go on smoother and stay on a lot longer than they did in the past. It just takes a little bit of practice. Use eyeliner along the lashline to give definition to the eyes and the illusion of fuller lashes. Use only on the outer corners to give the eye a gentle lift. Apply to the outer three-quarters of the lid for close-set eyes to draw the eyes out. (See page 40.)

Taylor's Tip

Eyeglass wearers often have a hard time with lashes hitting their lenses, making mascara or false eyelashes uncomfortable to wear. Look for shorter false lashes and curl them midway so that the tips bend up. This will prevent them from hitting the lens.

Taylor's Tip

To find your perfect eyelash strip length, first measure dry strips to the length of your eye, remove, and cut at the ends where necessary, then follow application directions.

Products and Tools

Pencil Liner

It's a good idea to spend a little extra for a quality eyeliner pencil. Avoid pencil liners that are waxy and hard, as they pull at the skin and don't deposit enough color. Pencils should be soft and go on smoothly. Smudge the line with an eyeliner brush and create a sultry, smoky eye. Set this liner with shadow to minimize bleeding, or use waterproof liner for defined lines that don't smudge or smear. Pencils are especially great to define the lower lashline.

Waterproof Liner

Most eyeliners of any type are available in waterproof form, which is great for women whose eyes tend to smear. The shape and skin type of some eyelids (namely oily lids, monolids, and some thin lids) are prone to smudging, particularly along the lower lashline. When investing in a waterproof liner, splurge on one that goes on smoothly and doesn't pull at the skin around the delicate eye area.

Colored Cream Liner

Liner comes in so many colors now, from bright pinks to metallic charcoal grays. Try it instead of eyeshadow to create a cleaner, smoky eye. Try it instead of powdered eyeshadow for a long-lasting, more intense eye. Since cream liner is heavier, it tends to last longer. Cream liners come in nice shimmers as well, which is great to create a dramatic look quickly. When using a vibrant color, add black or brown liner along the lashline to help neutralize the look. With colored liners, look for creamy textures that don't crumble or are too waxy or hard. If it glides on smoothly and stays put, it's a winner. If you find that cream liners smudge too easily, you might be better off with gel liners. (See page 39.)

Liquid Liner Brush

Liquid eyeliner is almost always found in a tube similar to mascara and comes with its own brush. Glide the tip of the brush along the lashline, pressing lightly for a thin line and increasing pressure for a thicker line. The newer brushes come in pen form with a brush at the tip. Clicking the pen allows the liquid to flow into the brush. These brushes tend to be shorter and easier to control.

Liquid Liner Foam

This dense foam liner is more forgiving than a brush and gives the control of a pencil, without losing the defined liquid liner look.

Gel Liner

This is a newcomer to the eyeliner world. I, like everyone else in the makeup business, was skeptical at first, but now I can't live without it. It's a great tool to create a perfect sharp line and also works well on mature skin because it gives the eye a lined look without pulling at the delicate skin. Apply it as quickly but as carefully as possible, as once it's set, it doesn't move.

Taylor's Tip

Monolids tend to be asymmetrical. Eyeliner can create the illusion of symmetry and add focal points and depth. If one eye is smaller than the other, make sure the eyeshadow closest to the lashline as well as the eyeliner are applied thicker when the eyes are closed so that when they are open, the shadow and eyeliner on both eyes appear even. Curling the lashes will make them appear fuller to add further symmetry.

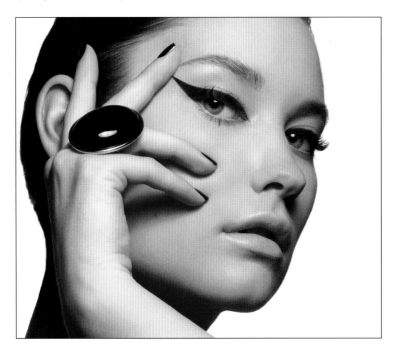

Application Methods

Corner Application

This soft daytime look is achieved by adding a little liner at the outer corners of the eye at a 45-degree angle and slightly extending the line to make eyes look wider and lifted.

Half Application

Apply eyeliner only on the outer half or three-quarters of the eye when trying to make close-set eyes appear wider. Here liner is applied thickly, creating more height.

Full Application

Applying eyeliner along the entire lashline is probably my favorite technique for a natural look that is still defined. Apply a thin line of black eyeliner on the upper lid as close to the lashline as possible. For close-set eyes, it's important to slightly extend the liner to draw the eyes farther out.

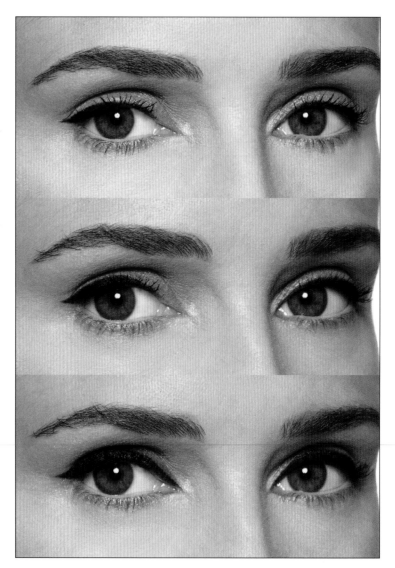

Using Eyeliner to Create Eye Shape

Having small eyes myself, for decades I've played around with eyeliner and learned how it can totally change the shape of the eye. Here are three examples of eyeliner tricks that quickly transform the eye.

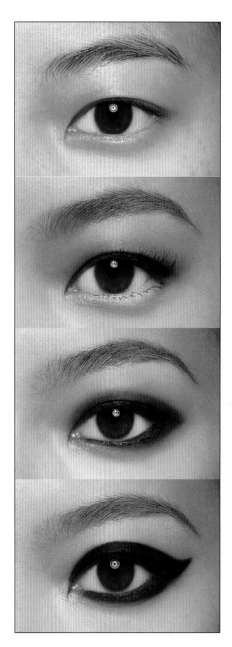

Upper Lid

Applying liner to the upper lashline only is one of the best ways to add height to the eyes. You can also extend liner out to give your eyes more length.

Smoky

Here eyeliner is applied on the upper and lower lashlines and blended out. As you can see, applying eyeliner around the entire eye won't make eyes appear smaller if the upper and lower lines are blended together.

Thick

Eyeliner application creates a focal point. Here eyes look larger and appear to be curved. Eyeliner helps create whatever shape you want to achieve.

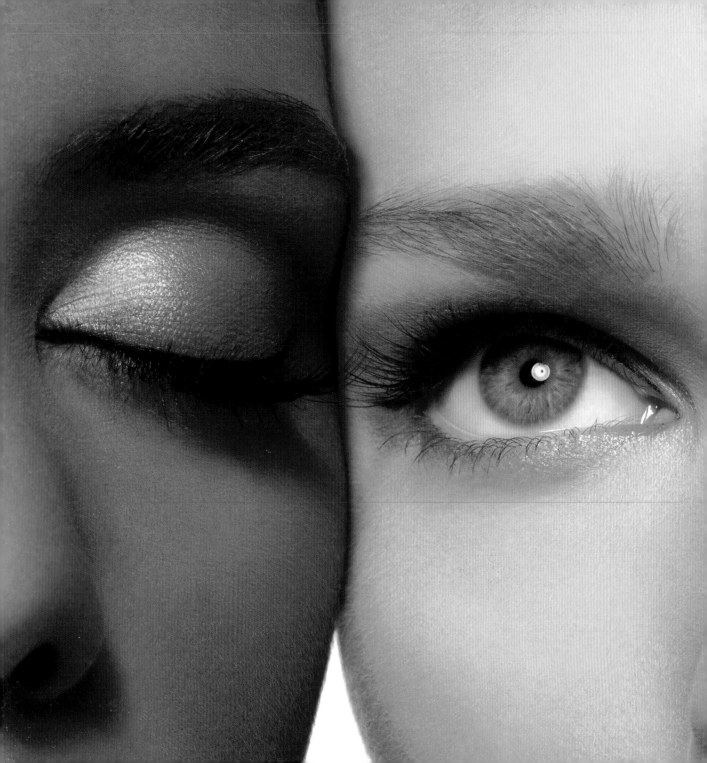

Eye Makeup Basics: Tips and Techniques for Every Shape and Color

It always surprises me when a woman feels as if she's the only one with a particular problem, such as, "I never know what color will look good on me" or "I have sensitive eyes." These are both common concerns. The important thing is to be educated about the appropriate products to address a specific issue and to learn why and how to use them. It will change your attitude toward makeup. In this chapter, you'll learn that not all eyeshadows are made the same, and you'll be given techniques on how to use them. Soon you'll be mixing and matching colors like a pro!

Put a Lid on It: Eyeshadow

No matter what challenges you've had with eyeshadows, whether it's sensitivity, creasing, or smearing, there is an eyeshadow out there for you. Technology has changed makeup greatly, eyeshadow included.

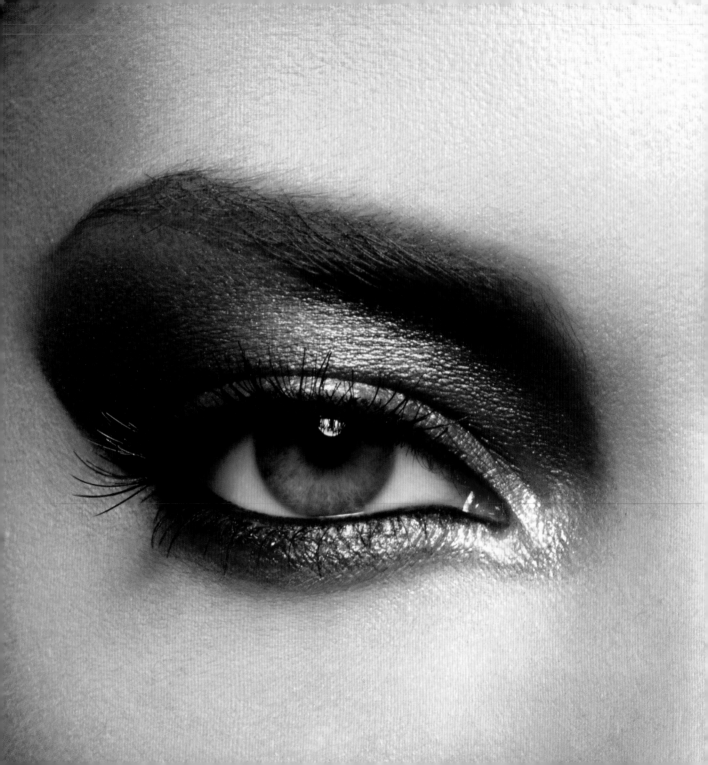

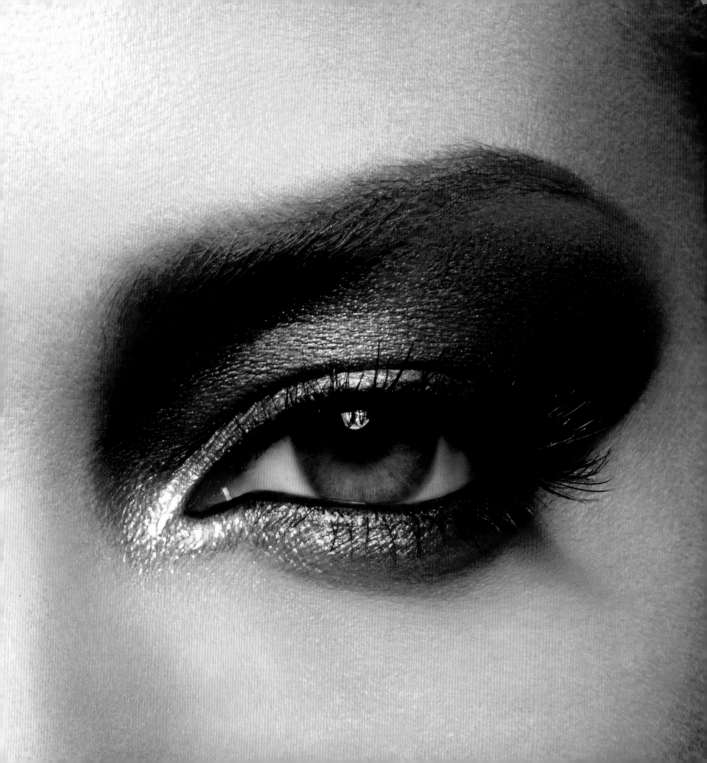

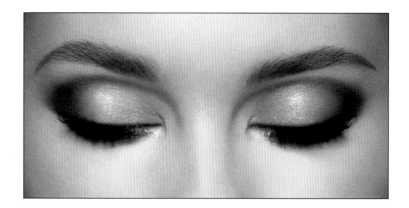

Many eyeshadows now even contain antioxidants—such as the anti-aging vitamins A, C, and E—and calming ingredients, such as green tea. And the color choices are endless—which can be a problem. Between endless color options, textures, and brands, there's a lot to think about when choosing an eyeshadow.

Product Guide

Eyeshadow Primers

Primers contain silicones and polymers that help eyeshadow stay in place. They are great if your eyeshadows have a tendency to crease and smudge or if you have very oily lids. Allow eye cream to dry before applying primer and apply it to bare skin (instead of foundation) for best results. If your challenge is discoloration, such as veiny lids, stick with foundation and powder to prime eyelids.

Cream-to-Powder Shadows

Cream-to-powder shadows start out as an easy-to-blend cream and set as a lighter powder, making them great for sheer application. Less prone to creasing than creams, these shadows are great for people who have oily lids but want the richer color of a cream shadow. Apply a powder shadow on top for even longer staying power.

Gel Shadows

Gel shadows are the newest technology of all the shadows. They can be used as liner or eyeshadow, come in more intense colors, and are great for highly dramatic looks. For best results, work with clean skin (no base, including foundation or concealer or primer on the lids). Gel shadows are also a great option if you have a lot of veins on the lid that must be covered. Avoid mixing powder eyeshadows with gels. Work fast with gel shadows, as once they set, the color doesn't move. Use with synthetic brushes or your ring finger and blend well for a more subdued look.

Pressed Shadows

Pressed shadows are the best for layering colors, and come in a dazzling array of colors and textures, from sheer shimmers to opaque matte black. There are even ones that contain green tea extracts and antioxidants. I prefer finely milled shadows that are silky and soft in texture. Avoid chalky textures that produce an uneven blend and can emphasize fine lines—the key word to avoid on an ingredient list is "calcium carbonate."

Stick Shadows

Stick shadows are cream shadows in stick form, but some do have a tendency to be a little denser in texture because of the way they are molded into shape. They seem to last longer than regular pot shadows (cream shadows usually found in small glass jars). Stick shadows are also great because they can be applied very quickly and without brushes. Great for makeup on the go!

Cream Shadows

Cream shadows are found in several types of packaging nowadays, from tubes, to wands, to pots. All produce great creamy looks, from sheer to opaque. The challenge with cream shadows is that they tend to smear and melt, often creasing on eyelids almost as soon as they are applied. Use sheerer colors to minimize the look of creasing, and avoid creams with too much shimmer, which will highlight fine lines. You may have to test a few before finding your perfect match. In drugstores, look for a key word such as "creaseless" and a great return policy, or go to your local makeup counter and test them out of tubes.

Loose Shadows

Loose shadows usually come in small jars and can be a little messy for the novice but offer a very precise application of color. They don't contain any binding agents, so they tend to be very light in texture. It's easy to inadvertently apply more color than intended with this type of shadow. For a more delicate look, use a small brush to apply highlighter loose shadow in white, opal, or gold to the inner corner of the eyes to open and brighten them. Then use a large brush and shake off excess powder for a beautifully soft application of pinks, golds, mauves, or pale purples.

Mineral Shadows

The mineral craze has created some die-hard fans, who swear by its apparent skin-improving qualities. Mineral powders only contain minerals, which means they don't contain any fancy extra ingredients and are limited in color. If you have challenges with blending, apply mineral shadows on a tissue or the back of your clean hand using an eyeshadow brush first before applying to eyelids. To make the shadow last, add base to your lids first.

Pure Pigments

Pure pigments come in loose shadow form and are very intense colors. All colors will most likely look their most vibrant in this form. They contain very few ingredients other than pigment, so they deliver more intense color than other eyeshadows. They're best for dramatic looks. For a fashion look or for a fun evening out, try wetting a shadow brush with water before applying to make the color even more intense. Try dark colors, such as brick, greens, and purples, or light colors, such as melon, gold, silver, or bronze, for added drama. Create a more natural look by

Taylor's Tip

Make sure that your brushes stay clean so that they don't collect bacteria. Use a mild detergent and water (I like to use shampoo or antibacterial washes) to wash brushes, similar to how you would wash your hair (but don't use conditioner!). Rinse thoroughly and lay brushes flat on a clean towel to dry. Don't sit them up in a cup when they're wet. The moisture coming down will loosen the glue that holds the hairs together. You can also use a brush cleaner (sold in beauty supply stores) to disinfect brushes quickly. In either case, make sure the brushes are thoroughly dry before use.

using a small amount of one shade and adding gradually to build to the desired effect. Remember, a little goes a long way.

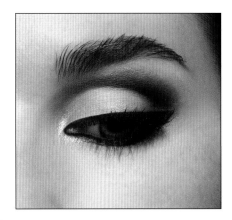

Brushes

Good-quality brushes should last ten years and are often what make the difference between a good eye makeup application and a great eye makeup application. I was once working with a celebrity who couldn't figure out why she didn't achieve such professional results when she did her own eye makeup at home. I asked to see her tools, and sure enough, she was using brow brushes for eyeliner and concealer brushes for eyeshadows. Eye makeup is an art and a science, and you need the proper tools to create the look you want.

Fluffy shadow brush

Great for looser, soft applications of shadow, such as applying a soft shimmer. Use it under the brow bone.

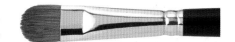

Small shadow detail brush

This is a multipurpose tool. Use it to highlight the inside corners of the eyes using shimmer, or as a thick eyeliner brush.

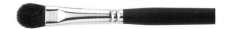

Large shadow brush

Use the flat side of this brush to apply heavier amounts of shadow onto the largest area on the lids. Apply eyeshadow with this brush by gently tapping the brush from side to side on the lid. Always use brushes made with soft hairs when working with the eye area; most of these brushes are made from goat or sable.

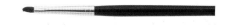

Small shadow contour brush

This brush is great for fine contouring of lids at the creases or for applying eyeshadow on the undereye area. It can also be used to smudge thicker amounts of eyeliner to create a dramatic look. (See page 72.)

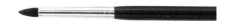

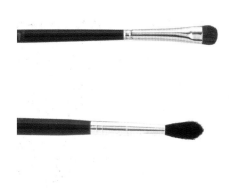

Small fluff shadow brush

Use to create a smoky effect on the eye. This brush is great for contouring lids at creases or putting darker shadows at the base of the lid only. (See "Monolids," page 56.)

Blend Brush

This is great to use to blend eyeshadows together. Be careful not to blend the different shadow layers too much, or the color will appear muddy. Remember: When you're dealing with the delicate eye area, it's important to buy a really soft brush with long, fine hairs.

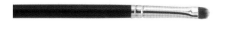

Flat Shadow Sponge Brush

Most people first learn to apply eyeshadow with a standard sponge brush because it often comes with the eyeshadow. It deposits heavy amounts of shadow to the eyelid. In the higher-end form, these brushes usually have disposable heads, so change them often.

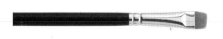

Liner Smudge Brush

This is a must-have for me. Use it to smooth jagged eyeliner to create an even line or smudge for a smoldering look. Look for short synthetic or sable bristles.

Flat Liner Brush

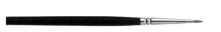

This brush is great for novices to apply liner on the lashline in sections. You can also create a lined look using eyeshadows. Try wetting the brush first to get more intense color. Because of its shape, it's also great for beginners who don't have the steadiest hands.

Liner Brush

Use this brush for creating a lined eye with gels or cream liners. I prefer the hairs to be semistiff for more control and ease.

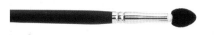

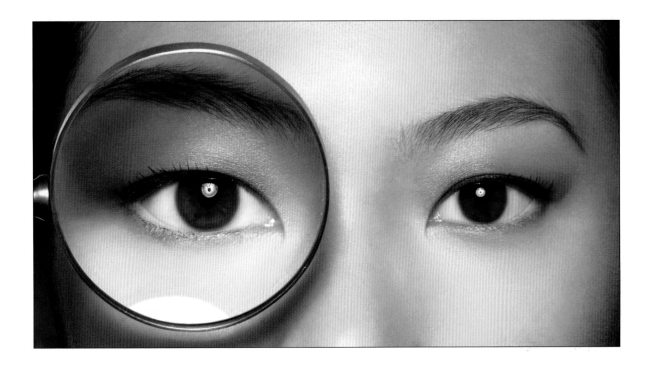

Working with Your Natural Shape

The following methods will show you how to apply eyeshadow colors to your specific eye shape in order to best flatter your eyes and face. Depending on your skin tone, substitute the appropriate foundations and concealers suitable for you.

Taylor's Tip

If you're looking for only a couple of essential brushes for most everyday makeup applications, the small fluff, detailed shadow brush, and large shadow brush can get you great results.

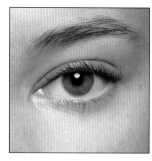

Upturned Eyes

While most women need to add lift to the outer corners of their eyes, upturned eyes have a natural lift at the corners, which can add an exotic feel to the face. To create balance to upturned eyes, apply shadow along the lower lashline, concentrating on the lower outer corner to help balance the eye and bring it down.

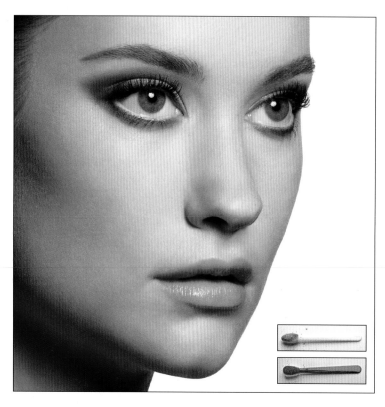

1. Apply light beige foundation to the eyelid and undereye.

2. Apply ivory concealer to the inner corner of the eye.

3. Set the foundation and concealer with translucent loose powder.

4. Apply gold eyeshadow to the base of the lid.

5. Apply dark brown eyeshadow along the top crease, outer corner, and lower lashline, concentrating on the lower outer corner.

6. Curl lashes and apply lengthening black mascara to the upper and lower eyelashes.

7. Apply short individual eyelashes along the upper lashline, alternating between short and long.

8. Apply light ash brown eyebrow powder, concentrating on the tail of the brow.

9. Apply clear brow gel.

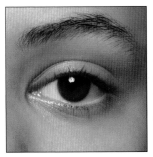

Downturned Eyes

Downturned eyes can look very sweet and innocent. The outer corners of the eyes angle down slightly, and a gentle soul seems to be peering through. To break away from this delicate look and add a little va va voom, apply eyeliner on the outer corners at a 45-degree angle to add lift.

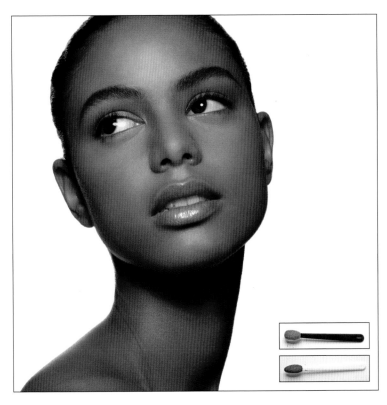

1. Apply honey foundation to the eyelid and undereye.

2. Apply light golden concealer to the inner corner and undereye.

3. Set the foundation and concealer with orange loose powder.

4. Apply taupe eyeshadow to the base of the lid and brow bone.

5. Apply warm brown eyeshadow to the outer corner to add lift to the eye.

6. Apply black pencil eyeliner on the outer upper corner. See corner application on page 40.

7. Curl lashes and apply full-volume black mascara to the upper and lower eyelashes.

8. Apply dark brown eyebrow pencil, with a lighter application at the beginning of the brow and a heavier application at the tail of the brow.

9. Apply clear brow gel.

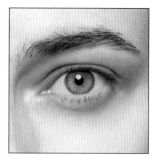

Thin Lids

Eyelids that have a thin fold (indentation) are between a monolid and a medium lid. When applying eyeshadows to thin lids, especially those that have large eyelid spacing (the space between the eye and the brow), it's best to work eyeshadows in layers as with monolids to create depth. (See page 56.)

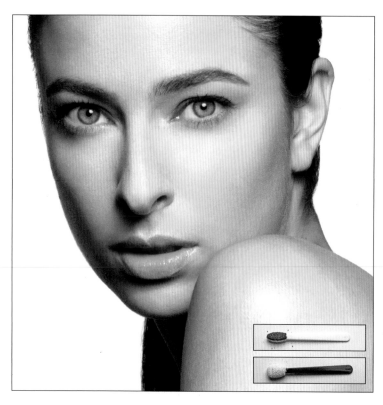

1. Apply beige foundation to the eyelid and undereye.

2. Apply light beige concealer to the inner corner of the eye.

3. Set the foundation and concealer with translucent loose powder.

4. Apply cool gray eyeshadow to the base of the lid and outer corner of the lower lid.

5. Apply white eyeshadow to the lower base of the lid close to the lashline, blending into the cool gray shadow.

6. Apply black cream eyeliner to the upper lid.

7. Curl lashes and apply volumizing black mascara to the upper and lower eyelashes.

8. Apply short and long individual eyelashes to the outer corner of the eye.

9. Apply dark ash brown eyebrow pencil, concentrating on the tail of the brow.

10. Apply clear brow gel.

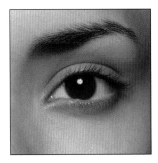

Medium Lids

If you have medium-size lids and even eyelid spacing, eye makeup application is going to be easier for you than for most others. Your eyelids are naturally defined, and shadows don't have to be placed in any intricate way to give you the illusion of balance. However, this can change with age, so make sure to take care of the lid area. You can apply eyeshadow in layers or accentuate the crease. It will all work on you.

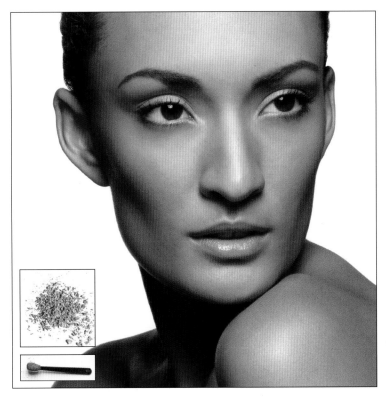

1. Apply warm beige foundation to the eyelid and undereye.

2. Apply ocher concealer to the inner corner and undereye.

3. Set the foundation and concealer with soft yellow loose powder.

4. Apply champagne eyeshadow to the base of the lid and inner corner of the eye.

5. Apply warm brown eyeshadow to the outer corner and along the crease.

6. Apply warm brown eyeshadow along the lower lashline.

7. Apply dark brown pencil eyeliner on the outer corner of the upper and lower lashlines.

8. Curl lashes and apply volumizing black mascara to the upper and lower eyelashes.

9. Apply dark brown eyebrow pencil, concentrating on the tail of the brow.

10. Apply clear brow gel.

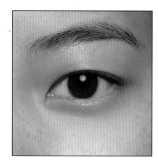

Monolids

Monolids are flat eyelids without a fold, which offer a lot of lid space to work with. To create depth, use the layering technique (see page 69), applying the darkest color closest to the lashline, neutral tones in the middle, and highlight colors at the brow bone. You can choose to apply one layer of shadow or layer up to four different shades (imagine colors directly on top of each other, similar to a rainbow, with the top color being the lightest and the bottom color being the darkest).

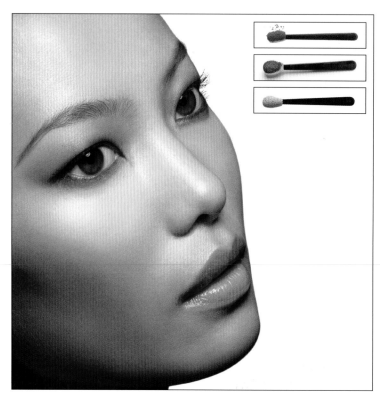

1. Apply warm beige foundation to the eyelid and undereye.

2. Apply beige concealer under the inner corner of the eye.

3. Set the foundation and concealer with translucent loose powder.

4. Apply mauve eyeshadow to the base of the lid.

5. Apply soft eggplant eyeshadow along the lashline, blending into the mauve eyeshadow.

6. Apply pale gold eyeshadow along the lower lashline, in the inner corner, and under the brow bone.

7. Apply black cream eyeliner along the upper lashline.

8. Curl lashes and apply waterproof black mascara to the upper and lower eyelashes.

9. Apply short and long individual eyelashes along the upper lashes.

10. Apply dark brown eyebrow pomade, using a synthetic angled brow brush, concentrating on slightly extending the tail of the brow.

11. Apply clear brow gel.

Taylor's Tip

This is also a great application for women with small eyes.

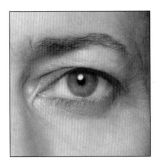

Hooded Lids

Hooded eyelids droop over the eye crease, pushing the eyelashes down over the eye. It can be frustrating to apply makeup, as products tend to smear, and eyeliner and eyeshadow applications disappear under the lid. When applying eyeshadow, add a contour color slightly above the hooded lid to create the illusion of depth and to draw the eyes up. Apply a thicker application of eyeliner, using a stay-put cream or gel eyeliner focusing on the outer corners of the eyes.

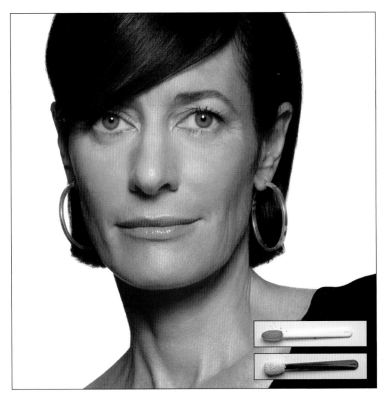

1. Apply sheer beige foundation to the eyelid and undereye.

2. Apply light beige cream concealer to the inner corner and undereye.

3. Set the foundation and concealer with translucent loose powder.

4. Apply golden taupe eyeshadow to the base of the lid, making sure to apply it more heavily at the outer corner and slightly above the crease.

5. Apply dark brown cream eyeliner in a 45-degree angle on the outer corner of the upper lashline. (See page 102.)

6. Curl lashes and apply black waterproof mascara to the upper and lower eyelashes to avoid smudging.

7. Add corner eyelashes to the outer corner to add additional lift to the eye.

8. Apply medium brown eyebrow pencil, concentrating on creating an arch to the brow and filling in the top and tail of the brow. (See page 103.)

9. Apply clear brow gel.

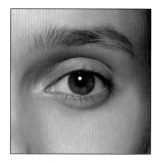

Deep-Set Eyes

Deep-set eyes are set farther back in the ocular bone. They are large and have a natural shadowing. Using dark shadows in the crease can make eyes appear even deeper. Apply lighter shadows above the crease to bring the crease forward. Using a shimmery shadow in melon, as shown, keeps deep-set eyes more neutral. If you want to apply a darker shadow, keep it closer to your lashline for the best effect.

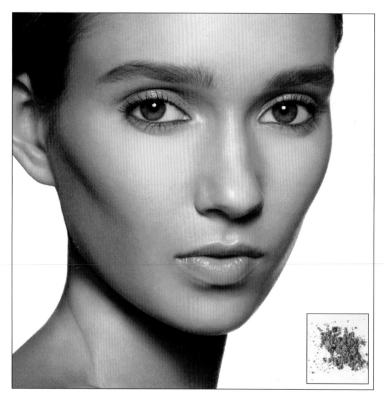

1. Apply warm beige foundation to the eyelid and undereye.

2. Apply ocher concealer to the inner corner and undereye.

3. Set the foundation and concealer with translucent loose powder.

4. Apply melon-colored pure pigment eyeshadow to the base of the lid.

5. Apply black waterproof eyeliner along the lower inside rim and outer corner of the upper lid.

6. Curl lashes and apply volumizing black mascara to the upper and lower eyelashes.

7. Apply light brown eyebrow pencil to the beginning of the brow.

8. Apply dark brown eyebrow pencil to the end of the brow.

9. Apply clear brow gel.

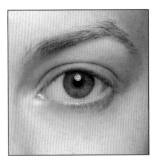

Large Eyes

Having large eyes and large lid space is a great perk, but be careful that your eyes don't overpower your whole face. To provide balance, keep dark shadows closer to the lashline and avoid going too far up to the brow.

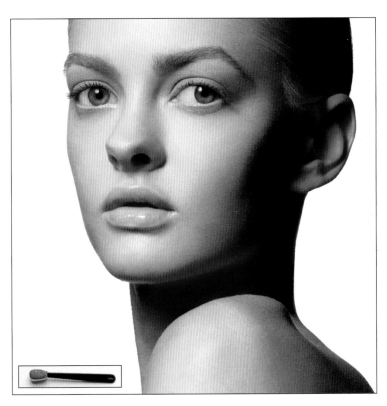

1. Apply pale beige foundation to the eyelid and undereye.

2. Apply ivory concealer to the inner corner of the eye.

3. Set the foundation and concealer with translucent loose powder.

4. Apply a slate eyeshadow to the entire base of the lid.

5. Curl lashes and apply lightly tinted black mascara to the upper lashes just to add a hint of color, making the shadow the focus.

6. Apply ash blond eyebrow pencil.

7. Apply clear brow gel.

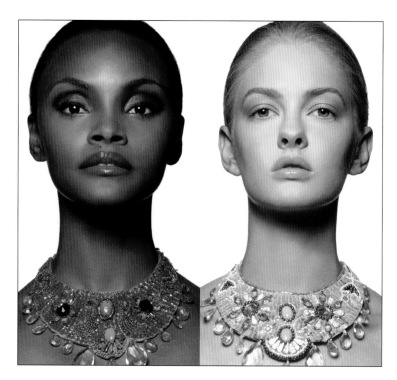

Working with Your Skin Tone

I have always believed that anyone can wear whatever color she wants as long as it suits her personality. However, it's important when choosing eye colors that you work with the right shade and tone for your skin.

Dark Skin

With darker skin, there are several factors to consider when choosing eyeshadows.

- Different shadow colors will play strongly off dark skin, with many colors appearing ashy. Colors such as white may appear gray on some dark skin. Look for light colors that have a little warmth. For example, pale yellow will cut ashiness and actually appear white against darker skin. (See page 80.)

■ When highlighting the eyelids, use colors lighter than your skin tone. Contour colors will add depth to the skin only if they are darker than your skin tone.

■ Soft colors with little pigment will not show up on the skin, which can be good to create a very natural look. Look for rich, heavily pigmented warm colors, such as gold, copper, bronze, berry, and eggplant, to create beautiful looks with added flair. When choosing colors to create more dramatic looks, work with bright pigmented colors, such as bright blue and pink. Choose hues and shades of color as opposed to tints. (See "Color Theory," page 64.)

■ Use rich black mascaras and eyeliners. Avoid gray eyeliners.

Pale Skin

Pale skin acts as a blank canvas. All colors appear more vibrant on pale skin, and dark colors can appear harsh and muddy. Dark grays can look like bruising if too much is applied.

■ Look for eyeshadows that are sheer and provide washes of color.

■ Try colors such as soft blue-gray, cool pink, taupe, and pale green.

■ Contour the eyes using colors only a few shades darker than your base shadow color, as contouring on pale skin shows up dramatically. Look for highlight colors that are lighter or equal to skin tone, such as white and opal. Highlight colors in shimmer form will appear more visible than a matte eyeshadow for pale skin.

■ When choosing bright eyeshadows, look for tints as opposed to shades (see "Color Theory," page 64) and apply them only on the base of the lid for a more natural effect.

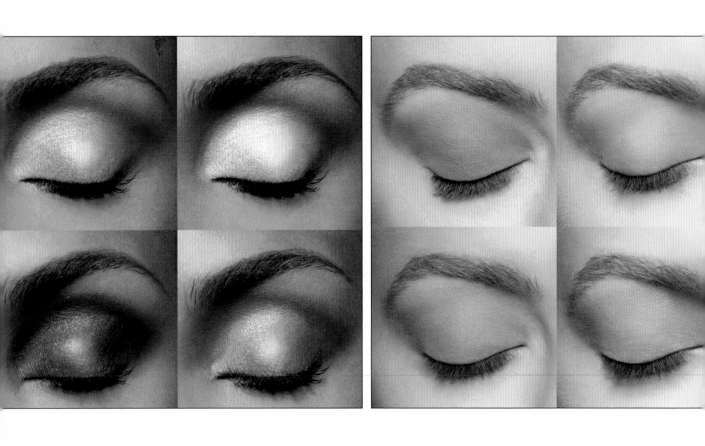

- Use softer eyeliner colors, such as brown or gray on pale skin. When using black, focus on the upper lid and avoid rimming the entire eye.
- For mascaras, try dark browns and soft blacks, which look more like dark gray for eyelashes.

Eyeshadow for Every Eye Color

The use of the right eyeshadows can bring out the color of the iris and intensify the beauty of the eyes. Look to the iris to see what different colors it contains, creating a harmonious look. For a more intense look, use colors farther from each other on the color wheel. For example, gold brings out the brightest in green eyes, and purple brings out the most in blue.

Brown

People with brown eyes have more choices of color than other iris colors, since brown is a neutral. Skin tone is a very important consideration when choosing color for brown eyes (see page 60). Brown eyes can be made to appear lighter by playing off the hints of gold and bronze found in most brown eyes. Wrapping eyeshadow color in the palest color of the iris around the entire eye can give the illusion of brighter-colored eyes. See other brown eye color looks on pages 83, 87, and 98.

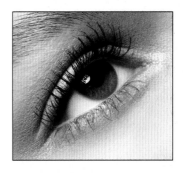

Blue

There are several variations of blue eyes, ranging from pale to deep blue. Here, blue eyes wrapped with a cool gray shadow appear to look gray. Pulling pale grays and silvers from the iris into makeup colors will intensify the eye's lightness, and wrapping the eye with black liner will create intense contrast, making the eyes look that much more intense. See other blue eye color looks on pages 76, 81, and 88.

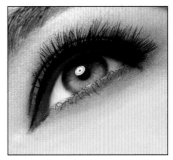

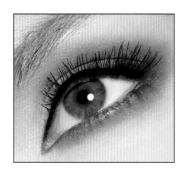

Green

Green irises can often appear blue depending on what colors are paired with them in clothes or on the face. Several shades can be seen in the iris, starting from the outside with forest green and fading into a pale green and hints of copper and dark brown near the pupil. Choosing the pale green around the eyes for a makeup color would intensify the lightness of the green. Here, I chose to create a natural eye using a warm brown, which is a darker version of the color near the pupil. See other green eye color looks on pages 88, 90, 91, 92, and 93.

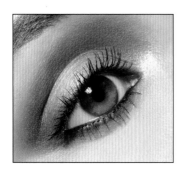

Hazel

Hazel eyes can look browner on some days and greener on others. Both colors are visible in the iris, along with gold tones. Try pulling pale greens and golds from the iris to make the eyes appear lighter and show off their colors. See other hazel eye color looks on pages 40, 58, 75, 79, 119, and 122.

Color Theory

Color can be a confusing subject, especially with the infinite amount of possibilities to choose from. Here's a little bit of basic color theory to help you choose the right color for you.

Understanding Color

Primary Color

All other colors are combinations of the primary colors, which are red, blue, and yellow. Black is a mixture of all the colors together and reflects no color, while white is an absence of color and reflects all colors.

What Is a Hue?

A hue is the true form of a color. While primary colors are really the only true colors, when we talk about hues, we are including the mixtures of primary colors. For example, mixing red with blue creates purple. While purple is not a true primary color, it is a true hue. For eye makeup, a hue will create the strongest form of color.

What Is a Tint?

A tint is made by adding white to any hue. This lightens the hue. Using green as an example, lime green would be a tint of green. For eye makeup, a tint will generally create a softer, more natural look, making the color more wearable. Light tints are used to bring out or highlight parts of the eye.

What Is a Shade?

A shade is a darker version of a hue—adding black instead of white. Forest green would be a shade of green. For eye makeup, a shade will generally create drama and add more depth wherever it is placed on the eye.

What Is a Tone?

A tone is a level of color—how light or dark a color is, rather than what actual color it is. The possibility of the number of tones that come out of one color is great. Lighter colors, such as yellow, will produce a smaller range of tones than a darker color, such as blue.

Monochromatic colors are a single hue or combinations of tones of a single hue. For example, different shades and tints of purple can be used together. Monochromatic color creates the most natural look when the tone levels are similar. For example, two lighter tones of a color would look more natural together on the eyelid than a light tone and a very dark tone of the color. I highly recommend this color scheme for creating depth and highlight for beginners. It's the simplest, and blending is easier to achieve. I also find it to be the prettiest. (See page 69.)

Taylor's Tip

A tint will highlight only if it is lighter than your skin tone. A shade will add depth only if it is darker than your skin tone.

COOL VS. WARM

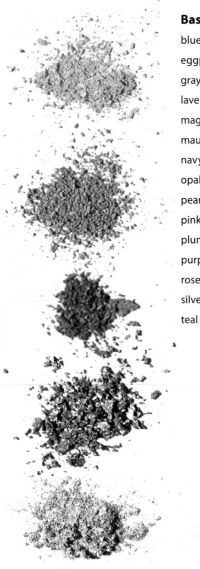

Basic Cool Colors

blue

eggplant

gray

lavender

magenta

mauve

navy

opal

pearl

pink

plum

purple

rose

silver

teal

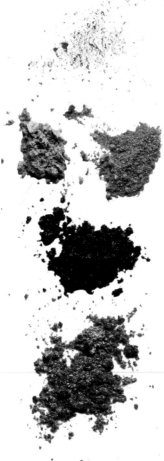

Basic Warm Colors

bronze

brown

chocolate

copper

coral

gold

honey

melon

mustard

orange

peach

red

some greens

tan

tangerine

taupe

yellow

Complementary colors are opposite each other on the color wheel. Complementary colors are actually more contrasting and will create more drama. They're called complementary colors because one color makes the other pop. Think about a Christmas tree—red balls on a green tree stand out the most. I highly recommend this color scheme for creating drama, and it is great for the makeup pro who wants to take eye makeup to the next level. It's more wearable if you use one color as an accent. For example, purple eyeshadow with gold shimmer on the inner corners of the eyes is actually very wearable yet complementary. (See page 78.)

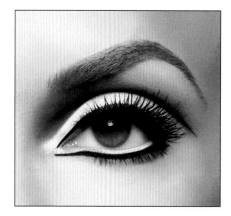

Analogous colors are colors that are next to each other on the color wheel. Blue and purple would be analogous colors. While analogous colors aren't as contrasting as complementary colors and are therefore more wearable, they are still quite dramatic. Try one color in shimmer form and the other in matte to create dimension and soften the look. Purple shimmer at the base of the lid with blue shadow lined along the lashline would work better than an entire lid of half-purple and half-blue shadow. (See page 97.)

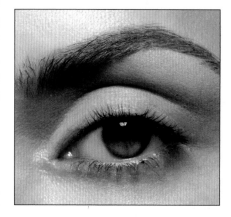

Understanding Dark and Light

Colors that are lighter in tone than your skin tone will create highlight, bringing forward that part of your eye. Colors that are darker than your skin tone will create depth and contouring, causing that part of your eye to appear to recede.

Drama happens when there is significant difference in the level of highlight and shadow. Here the highlight color (silver) is significantly lighter than the model's skin tone. (This makes the contrast even starker.) The shadow colors (navy and black) are much darker than her skin tone. Using contrasting tones of a color (such as navy blue and light blue) will also create a dramatic effect.

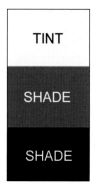

TINT

SHADE

SHADE

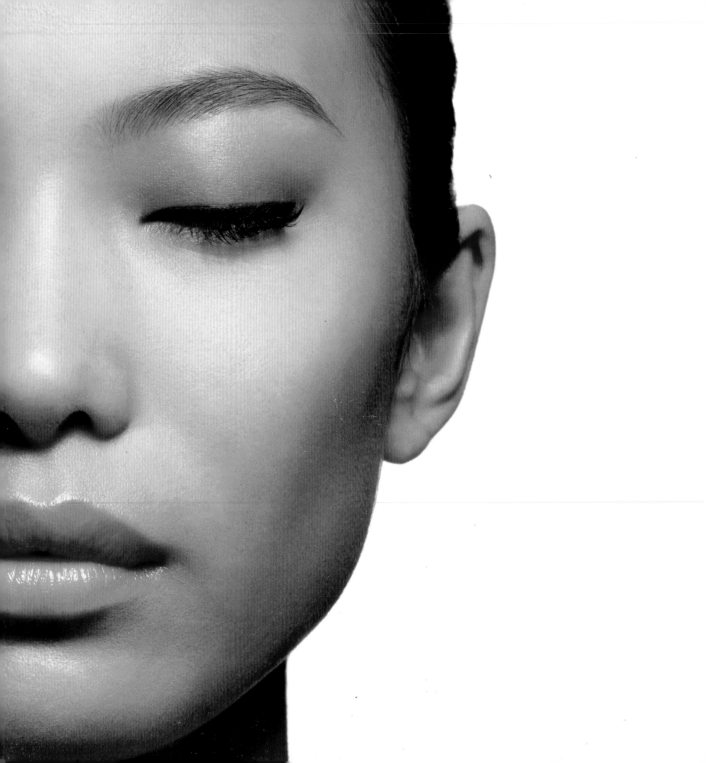

Eyeshadow Techniques

Layering

Layering is applying eyeshadow on a gradient, with the lightest shadow color under the brow bone and the darkest color along the lashline. This technique is great for any makeup novice and essential for people with monolids as well as thin lids. You can layer up to four shades, ending with a layer of eyeliner.

1. Apply warm beige foundation to the eyelid and undereye.

2. Apply beige concealer under the inner corner of the eye.

3. Set the foundation with translucent loose powder.

4. Apply soft rose eyeshadow to the base of the lid (Step 1).

5. Apply deep rose eyeshadow along the lashline, blending into the soft rose eyeshadow (Step 2).

6. Apply pale pink eyeshadow along the lower lashline, in the inner corner, and under the brow bone (Step 3).

7. Apply black cream eyeliner along the upper lashline (Step 4).

8. Curl lashes and apply waterproof black mascara to the upper and lower eyelashes.

9. Apply short and long individual eyelashes along the upper lashes.

10. Apply dark brown eyebrow pomade, concentrating on the tail of brow.

11. Apply clear brow gel.

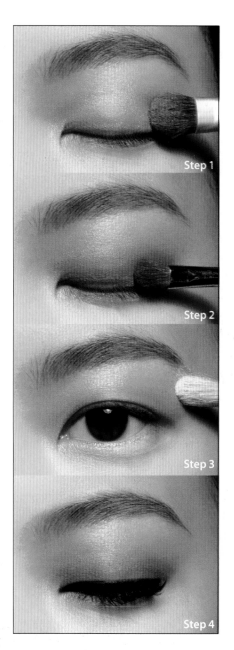

Step 1

This is the base of the lid, the largest section of the eye area. The shadow applied here will be the most visible as well as the base color. Work other colors around this base to highlight or add depth to the eyes. When

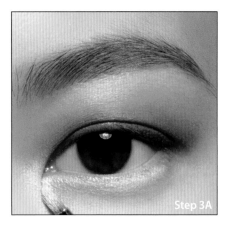

Step 3A

applying eyeshadow in this section alone, use a neutral tone. Think of soft, warm colors, such as taupe or mauve. This creates a very natural daytime look. As shown, start the shadow at the base of the lashes and blend up.

Step 2

This is the contour layer of eyeshadow that adds depth to the eye. When applied using the layering technique, this layer of eyeshadow is closest to the eyeliner layer. For contouring eyes (see page 71) with a fold, this layer is added in the crease as well as the outer corner of the lid to add depth. Adding this section of eyeshadow helps define the shape of the eye. For every day, choose colors that are darker versions of the base color, but dark browns, grays, and black shadows can also be used for a darker smoky effect.

Step 3

This is the brow bone area. Using a light shimmer or light matte tone accentuates the brow bone. Use light opal tones when working with cool shadow colors and light gold tones when working with warm colors. (See "Color Theory," page 64.) Use off-white or pale yellow tones for a more natural highlight. When using this layer alone, go from the brow bone and blend all the way to the lashline.

Step 3A

This is the inner corner of the eye. Add a little lighter color here to open up and brighten the eye.

Step 4

This last layer adds definition to the eye and is applied along the lashline. It typically consists of dark eyeliners in dark brown, gray, or black. During the day, apply a thin line for a more natural look.

Taylor's Tip

Use highlight eyeshadows on the inner corners of the eyes to open up and brighten the eyes. For wide-set eyes, use dark eyeliner along the entire upper lashline to draw the eyes closer together.

Taylor's Tip

For a smoky evening look or a stronger daytime look, apply brighter colors, such as pinks, purples, greens, and even blues. Add other colors to warm up or make the look dramatic.

Undereyes

When applying makeup under the eyes, continue to work in layers, mirroring the upper lid application. (See page 72.) For a daytime look, use only on the lower outer corners of the eyes, or use only one or two colors.

Contouring Eyelids

Contouring is arguably the most widely used of all eyeshadow application techniques. It's the technique that most makeup artists are trained to use, and it has become popular with the general public. It's great for adding depth to creases and opening up the eye. Women without an eyelid crease should use the layering technique instead.

Taylor's Tip

If you have small eyes, apply Steps 2 and 4 thicker and slightly outside the natural upper lashline to give length and height to your eyes.

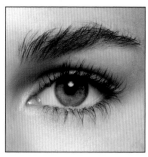

Step-by-Step Smoky

The smoky eye has gotten a bad wrap. A smoky eye should be sultry, nicely blended—a stronger look but still clean and sexy. Darker shadows should be used, but avoid the dreaded "raccoon eyes"—this color palette is not limited to blue or gray shadows. I actually prefer to create smoky eyes using bronzes, plums, and browns.

Once you break down *how* to create a smoky eye into steps, it's really quite easy to execute. It's only a matter of filling in the appropriate shadow colors in the right order. Pair this eye with a neutral lip to make a fashion statement. Use tones of one color to create a sultry natural daytime look.

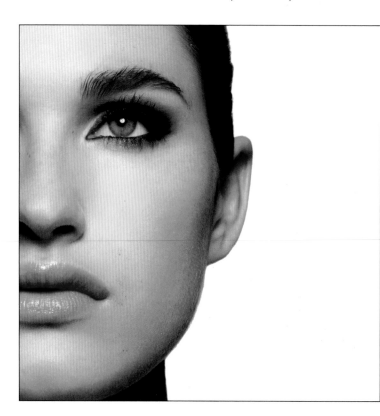

STEP 1
Here we started with white on the base of the lid.

STEP 2
Adding this section of eyeshadow creates contour and depth. Add soft blue eyeshadow in a triangle shape to add depth to the lid.

STEP 3
Add black shadows for a darker smoky effect. For a more natural look, try a medium gray shadow. When contouring, darker colors should be applied in the crease of the eyelid to add depth. You can also apply it along the outer crease as well as the outer corner of the eye.

STEP 4
For a dark smoky eye, black eyeliner is always a good choice, but you can swap it out for something more subtle or neutral and use brown or gray liner. Liner can give the illusion of thicker lashes and add depth. It can also be used to emphasize or change the shape of the eye. (See page 41.)

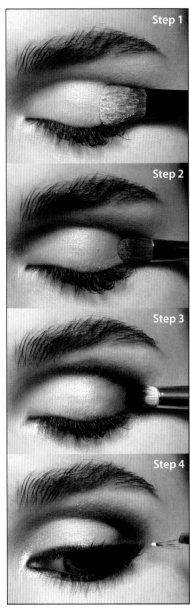

Upper Lid Application

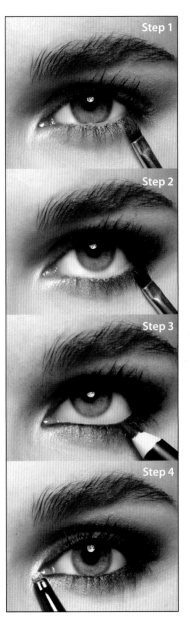

Undereye Application

Undereye Application

When applying eyeshadow under the eye, mirror the technique from the upper lid to add symmetry and a little more drama, especially for a smoky eye.

STEP 1
Apply soft blue eyeshadow along the lower lashline.

STEP 2
Apply black eyeshadow to the lower outer corner for a sultry effect.

STEP 3
Apply eyeliner to the inner rim of the eye. This can also be applied along the lashline if you prefer.

STEP 4
Apply a highlight color to the inner corner to add softness and a little sparkle to a dark smoky eye.

Taylor's Tips

Black eyeliner inside the lower rims of the eyes creates an instantly sexy look. For a softer version, try dark brown or gray.

Clean up stray eyeshadow using cotton swabs and eye makeup remover or eye cream, and apply face makeup afterward.

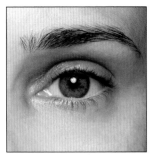

Classic Smoky

This traditional application method uses black eyeliner to achieve an even more dramatic effect.

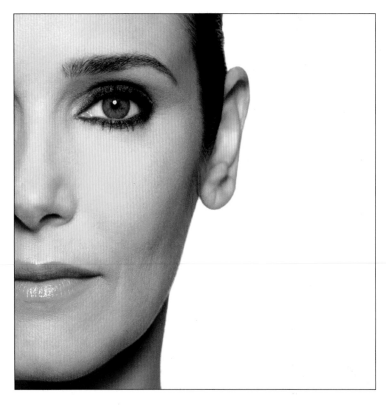

1. As with any eyeshadow application, start with a foundation and powder to prime the eyelid.

2. Apply a warm neutral shadow over the base of the lid.

3. Using a pencil eyeliner, apply black eyeliner along the upper lashline.

4. Using a pencil eyeliner, apply black eyeliner along the lower lashline.

5. Use the same black eyeliner and line inside the lower rim.

6. Using a liner smudge brush and black eyeshadow, smudge the upper and lower eyeliner by wiggling the brush side to side to create a smoky effect.

7. Apply white shimmer shadow in the inner corner for added glamour (optional).

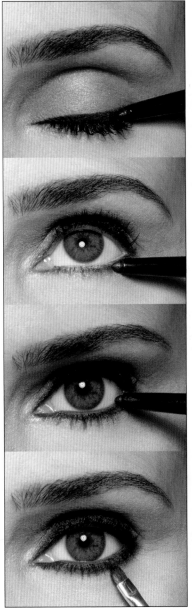

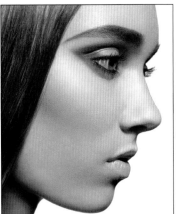

The Extras

THE EXTENSION

The extension is a method of pulling the outer corners of shadow and/or liner closer to the temples so that the eyes are lengthened. Make it look natural by using light colors and extending eyeshadow only slightly; or create a dramatic look by using dark eyeshadows and elongating to make it more fantasy. This technique is popular on the runway.

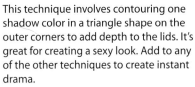

THE TRIANGLE

This technique involves contouring one shadow color in a triangle shape on the outer corners to add depth to the lids. It's great for creating a sexy look. Add to any of the other techniques to create instant drama.

THE ARCH

The arch involves placing contour eyeshadow along the entire crease. This is a great technique to open up the eyes. Creating a < and > shape at the outer corners finishes the arch more dramatically. Here we used an eyeshadow a few shades darker than the skin tone to create an arch that looks perfectly natural.

Classic Smoky Application

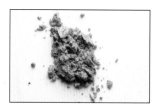

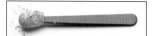

Multicolor Eyeshadow

Multiple shades of color on the lid can be a great way to experiment with color and create fun looks for the adventurous. Use cream or powder eyeshadows in the same soft tones to create a glow.

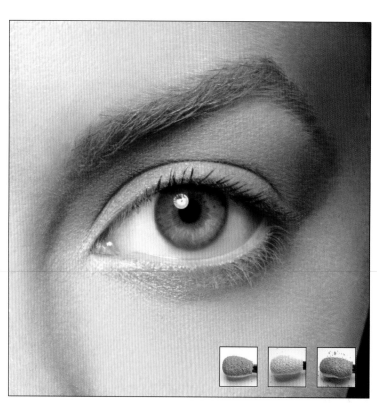

1. Apply pale beige foundation to the eyelid and undereye.

2. Apply ivory concealer to the inner corner of the eye.

3. Set the foundation and concealer with translucent loose powder.

4. Apply pink eyeshadow to the first third of the lid (starting at the inner corner), angling toward the center.

5. Apply matte gold shadow to the middle of the eyelid.

6. Apply matte warm green shadow to the outer third of the lid, slightly extending up to the eyebrow.

7. Apply gold shadow along the lower lashline.

8. Apply pale gold shimmer shadow to the inner corner of the eye.

9. Curl lashes and apply lightly tinted black mascara to the upper lashline just to add a hint of color to the lashes, making shadow the focus.

10. Apply ash blond eyebrow powder, concentrating on the tail of the brow.

11. Apply clear brow gel.

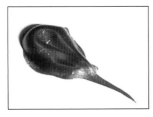

Gold Cream

Using opaque cream eyeshadows feels like painting. This thick shadow glides over the lid as richly as an oil paint. Owing to the intensity of cream shadows, using just one color on the base of the lid is much more forgiving than multiple colors and is very wearable. Notice how the look is very simple but still highly dramatic.

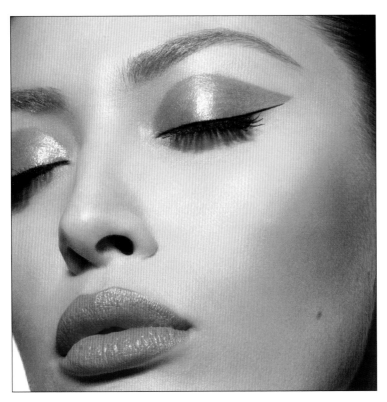

1. Apply beige foundation to the eyelid and undereye.

2. Apply light beige concealer to the inner corner and undereye.

3. Apply gold-colored cream eyeshadow to the base of the lid, creating a sharp point at the end of the lid.

4. Apply a thin line of black liquid eyeliner along the upper lashline, extending slightly outside the lashline.

5. Curl lashes and apply lengthening mascara to the upper and lower eyelashes.

6. Apply a full eyelash strip to the upper lashline.

7. Fill in the brow with light ash brown eyebrow powder.

8. Apply gold eyebrow gel.

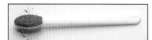

Violet

If you've always stuck with brown shades, try graduating to a warm violet color. Violet shadow against green eyes gives a radiant contrast that looks alluring. The color looks good on anyone, from fair to dark skin, young or old. Don't apply much; just a sheer wash will add a little oomph to a makeup look. In this image, the violet has iridescence in it that adds shimmer to the eyes.

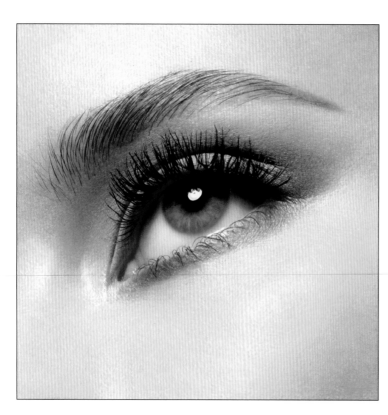

1. Apply light beige foundation to the eyelid and undereye.

2. Apply ivory concealer to the inner corner of the eye.

3. Set the foundation and concealer with translucent loose powder.

4. Apply honey eyeshadow to the base of the lid.

5. Apply violet eyeshadow along the crease, outer corner, and lower lashline.

6. Curl lashes and apply lengthening black mascara to the upper and lower eyelashes.

7. Apply a short eyelash strip along the upper lashline.

8. Apply medium brown eyebrow pencil, concentrating on the tail of the brow.

9. Apply clear brow gel.

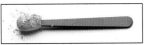

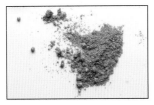

Bright

Bright eyeshadows can make the eyes look dramatic with a single swipe of color. Here a layer of light gold illuminates the eyes and draws attention instantly. When using bright eyeshadows, it's best to stick with only one color on the base of the eyelid. Black liner and lashes break the color at the lashline and keep the look defined and pretty.

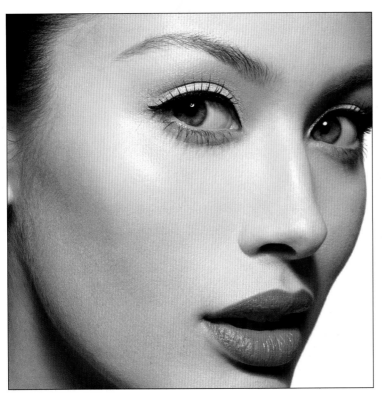

1. Apply beige foundation to the eyelid and undereye.

2. Apply light beige concealer to the inner corner and undereye.

3. Apply bright yellow pure pigment eyeshadow to the base of the lid, creating a sharp point at the end of the lid.

4. Apply a thin line of black liquid eyeliner along the upper lashline, extending slightly outside the eye and lifting the end at a 45-degree angle.

5. Curl lashes and apply lengthening mascara to the upper and lower eyelashes.

6. Apply a full eyelash strip to the upper lashline.

7. Apply light ash brown eyebrow powder to brow.

8. Apply gold brow gel.

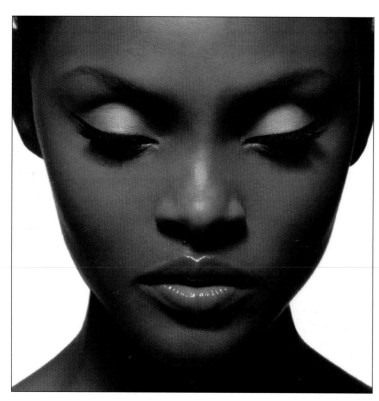

White

White eyeshadow instantly highlights eyes. On dark skin, pale yellow appears white. True white on dark skin can turn gray, so when using light colors on dark skin, it's important to choose colors that contain a slight pink or yellow undertone. Paired with winged eyeliner, this creates an instant high-fashion look. To make the look more wearable for the day, apply black eyeliner only on the upper lid, and minimize the lift of the winged line.

1. Apply chestnut stick foundation to the eyelid and undereye.

2. Apply golden brown concealer to the inner corner and undereye.

3. Set the foundation and concealer with orange loose powder.

4. Apply pale yellow eyeshadow to the base of the eyelid.

5. Apply a thin line of black cream eyeliner along the upper lashline, extending up and out.

6. Apply a thin line of black cream eyeliner to the outer corner of the lower lashline and extend out parallel with the upper lid eyeliner.

7. Apply white eyeliner on the inner corner of the upper and lower lashline.

8. Curl lashes and apply volumizing mascara to the upper and lower eyelashes.

9. Apply a short eyelash strip to the entire upper lashline and add a few long individual eyelashes to the upper outer corner.

10. Apply dark brown eyebrow pomade.

11. Apply clear brow gel.

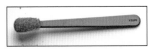

Bold Bronze

Most women can wear bronze well. It's one of those colors that illuminates the eyes and adds a hint of sexiness. It brings out the best in green and blue eyes, creating a beautiful contrast, and makes brown eyes brighter. It's great for light to dark skin tones and every shade in between. For pale skin, use only a light wash and wear it close to the lashline.

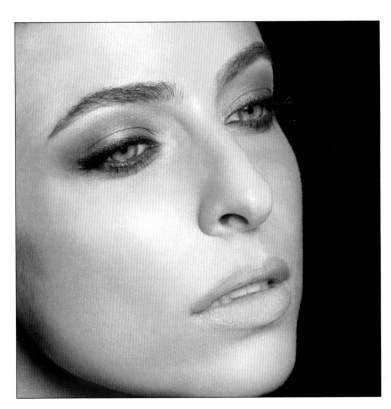

1. Apply beige foundation to the eyelid and undereye.

2. Apply light beige concealer to the inner corner of the eye.

3. Set the foundation and concealer with loose golden shimmering powder.

4. Apply bronze eyeshadow to the base of the lid and around the entire eye, slightly extending the outer corner.

5. Apply black cream eyeliner to the upper lid.

6. Curl lashes and apply black mascara to the upper and lower eyelashes.

7. Apply short and long individual eyelashes to the outer corner of the eye.

8. Apply dark ash brown eyebrow pencil.

9. Apply clear brow gel.

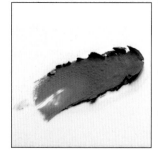

Vibrant Blue

Bright blue cream eyeshadow has been around since the fifties and adds instant color without needing too much product. Here eyes are lined to have a more period feel, but you can make the look more wearable by simply applying a thinner coat of blue cream eyeshadow at the base of the lid and black liner only along the upper lashline. This look is also great for those who have dark olive skin tones.

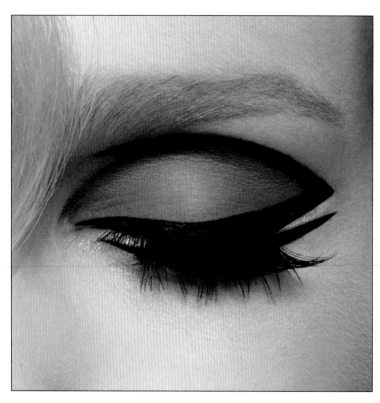

1. Apply beige foundation to the eyelid and undereye.

2. Apply beige concealer to the inner corner of the eye.

3. Apply bright blue cream shadow at the base of the lid.

4. Apply black cream eyeliner to the upper lid, winging the line up and out.

5. Apply black cream eyeliner inside the entire crease while looking down. Be careful not to look up until the liner has dried completely (about thirty seconds).

6. Apply black eyeliner along the lower lashline, extending and winging the line up to be parallel with the line of the upper lid.

7. Apply white eyeliner between the black lines and on the inside rim of the lower lashes.

8. Curl lashes and apply black mascara to the upper and lower eyelashes.

9. Apply thick chunks of short and long individual eyelashes along the upper lashline, with the longest on the outer corner of the eye.

10. Apply short individual lashes along the lower lashline.

11. Apply blond eyebrow pencil.

12. Apply clear brow gel.

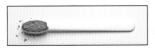
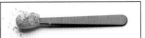

Apple Green

I find inspiration everywhere. Even the simple green apple has different colors in it, which flow continuously from light to dark. A shimmering green looks beautiful on honey skin tones, but the color is wearable on almost everyone, no matter what your skin tone or age.

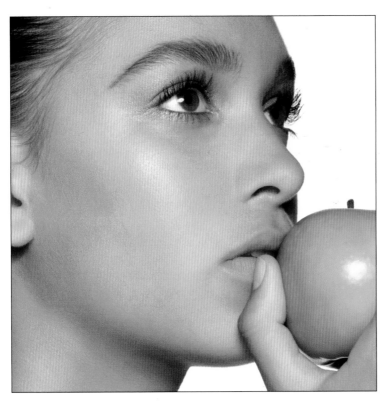

1. Apply light honey foundation to the eyelid and undereye.

2. Apply ochre concealer to the inner corner of the eye.

3. Set the foundation and concealer with medium warm beige loose powder.

4. Apply shimmering green eyeshadow on the base of the lid, applying above the crease but not under the brow bone. Extend the shadow to wing out.

5. Apply the same shimmering green eyeshadow along the lower lashline.

6. Apply a golden lemon shimmer loose powder eyeshadow on the inner corner of the eye.

7. Curl lashes and apply volumizing black mascara to the upper and lower eyelashes.

8. Apply dark brown eyebrow pencil, focusing on the outer two-thirds of the brow.

9. Apply clear brow gel, brushing up to create a full look.

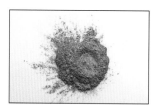

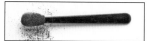

Metallic

Metallic eyeshadow adds instant glam to any makeup look. It gives eyes a very rock star feel. Great for an evening out at the club, it's also workable during the day in lighter applications—unless, of course, you *are* a rock star or at least want to look like one.

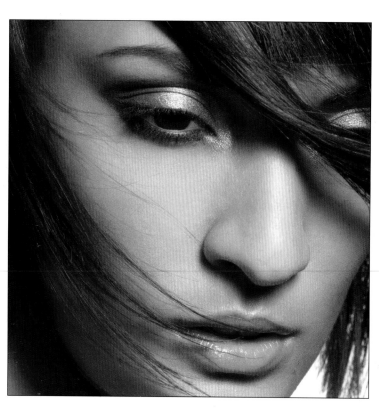

1. Apply honey foundation to the eyelid and undereye.

2. Apply ocher concealer to the inner corner and undereye.

3. Set the foundation and concealer with light shimmering loose powder.

4. Apply gold metallic eyeshadow pigment to the base of the lid and inner corner of the eye.

5. Apply dark brown eyeshadow to the outer corner and along the crease.

6. Apply dark brown eyeshadow along the lower lashline.

7. Apply dark brown pencil eyeliner on the inside of the inner rim and blend onto the lower lashline.

8. Curl lashes and apply volumizing black mascara to the upper and lower eyelashes.

9. Apply medium brown eyebrow pencil, concentrating on the tail of the brow.

10. Apply clear brow gel.

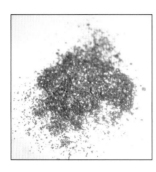

Glitter

There is no better way to add sparkle than glitter eyeshadow. It gives the look of glitter without too much sparkle or discomfort. This look will definitely turn more than a few heads. For the most natural look, use a glitter shade that is close to your skin tone.

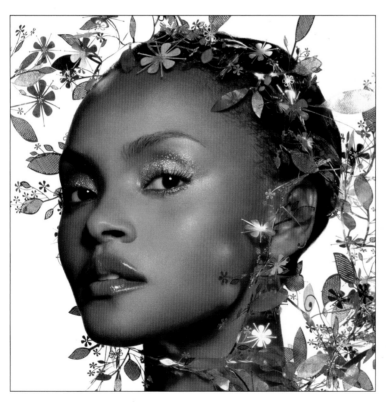

1. Apply chestnut stick foundation to the eyelid and undereye.

2. Apply golden brown concealer to the inner corner and undereye.

3. Set with orange powder.

4. Apply bronze glitter eyeshadow to the base of the eyelid.

5. Apply black eyeliner in the inside rim of the lower lid.

6. Curl lashes and apply black volumizing mascara to the upper and lower eyelashes.

7. Apply short and long individual eyelashes to the outer corner of the eye.

8. Apply dark brown eyebrow pomade.

9. Apply clear brow gel.

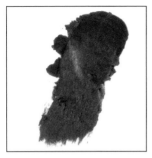

Dark and Glossy

Possibly one of the most dramatic eye looks, this one is for the adventurous and bold. To make the look more wearable, apply shadows closer to the lashline, giving it more of a smoky gloss effect.

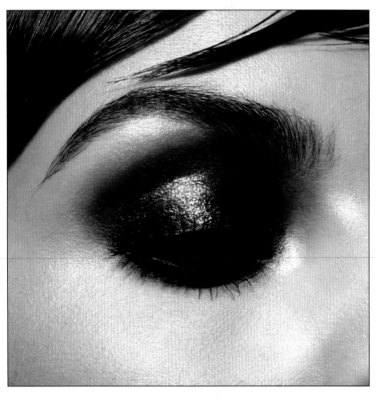

1. Apply beige foundation to the eyelid and undereye.

2. Apply beige stick concealer to the inner corner and undereye.

3. Set the foundation and concealer with translucent loose powder.

4. Apply dark bronze cream eyeshadow to the base of the lid, extending out and along the lower lashline.

5. Apply black cream eyeliner along the upper lashline and blend gently into the bronze cream.

6. Apply black cream eyeliner along the lower lashline.

7. Apply black pencil eyeliner inside the lower rim.

8. Curl lashes and apply black mascara to the upper and lower eyelashes.

9. Apply a full eyelash strip to the upper lashline.

10. Gently apply clear eyegloss on top of the cream shadow at the center of the lid.

11. Apply dark brown eyebrow pomade.

12. Apply clear brow gel.

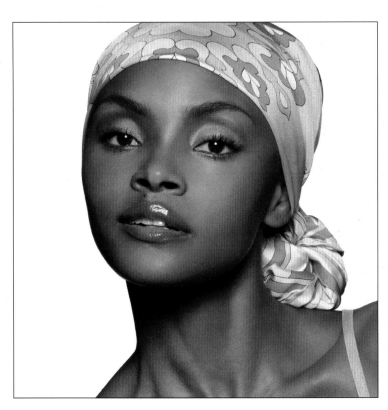

Tie It Up

When choosing an eyeshadow color, it is important to consider not only skin tone or eye color but also accessories. Pull colors from accessories that are close to the face, such as scarves, hats, and earrings. Here the base color of the scarf, a warm pink, is the inspiration for applying a darker version of it with shimmer to highlight the eyes.

1. Apply chestnut stick foundation to the eyelid and undereye.

2. Apply golden brown concealer to the inner corner and undereye.

3. Set the foundation and concealer with orange powder.

4. Apply warm pink shimmery eyeshadow to the base of the lid and above the crease.

5. Apply black eyeliner in the inside rim of the lower lid.

6. Curl lashes and apply black volumizing mascara to the upper and lower eyelashes.

7. Apply dark brown eyebrow pomade.

8. Apply clear brow gel.

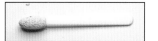
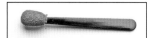

Tie It In

When wearing a "statement piece," such as this bold-colored hat, choose your focal point and avoid fighting the colors. Here a warm plum shadow allows eye makeup to blend well with the accessory but not overpower it.

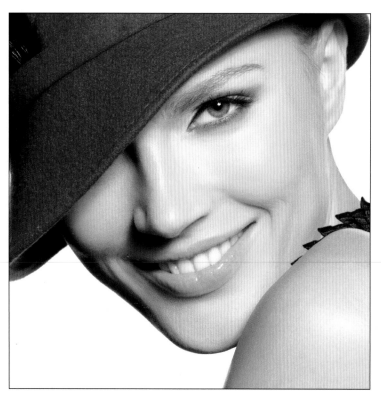

1. Apply beige foundation to the eyelid and undereye.

2. Apply beige stick concealer to the inner corner and undereye.

3. Set the foundation and concealer with translucent loose powder.

4. Apply matte white eyeshadow to the base of the lid, along the inner corner, and under the brow bone.

5. Apply warm plum eyeshadow along the top crease and softly along the lower lashline, connecting the shadow at the outer corner.

6. Curl lashes and apply black mascara to the upper and lower eyelashes.

7. Apply short and long individual eyelashes to the corner of the eye.

8. Apply ash blond eyebrow powder.

9. Apply clear brow gel.

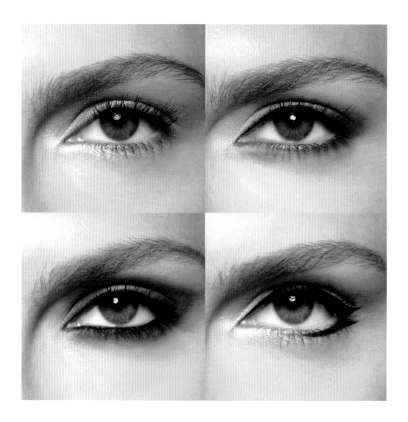

One Eye Four Ways

Your eye makeup should reflect your mood and attitude. It can also make a difference in how you are perceived. You can be whomever you want to be, whether it's daring, natural, classic, or sultry. When creating these looks, balance is essential to making them wearable. If your eye makeup is dark, stick with neutral lips; if your lip color is dark, keep your eyes neutral; and so on.

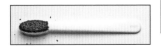
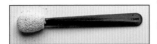

Daring

Take a little risk when applying eye makeup. You don't have to make drastic changes; simply winging out your liner a little higher can add just the right amount of drama.

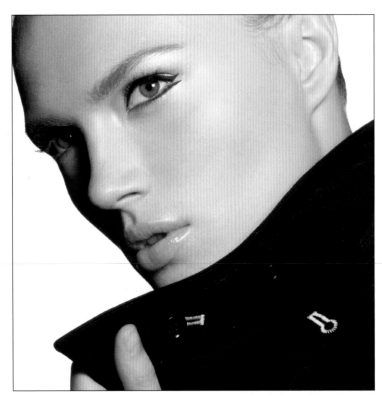

1. Apply beige foundation to the eyelid and undereye.

2. Apply beige stick concealer to the inner corner and undereye.

3. Set the foundation and concealer with translucent loose powder.

4. Apply cool gray eyeshadow to the base of the lid.

5. Apply white eyeshadow to the brow bone.

6. Using an eyeliner brush, apply black cream eyeliner along the upper lashline and extend at a 45-degree angle.

7. Apply black cream eyeliner along the outer half of the lower lashline, extending out and making sure not to connect with the upper lashline.

8. Curl lashes and apply black mascara to the upper and lower eyelashes.

9. Apply short and long individual eyelashes, alternately, to the outer corner of the eye.

10. Apply ash blond eyebrow powder.

11. Apply clear brow gel.

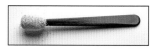
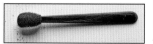

Natural

For clean yet defined looks, use neutral shadows, with not too much shimmer or color. Use colors only a few shades darker than your natural skin tone—stick with taupes, mauves, and browns. I have yet to meet a woman this look didn't work on.

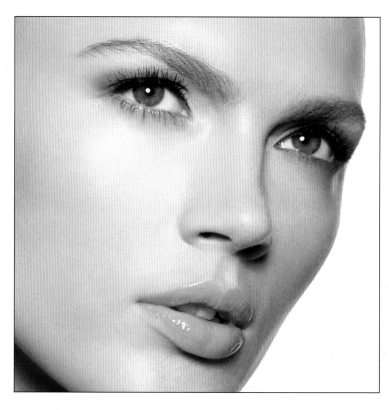

1. Apply beige foundation to the eyelid and undereye.

2. Apply beige stick concealer to the inner corner and undereye.

3. Set the foundation and concealer with translucent loose powder.

4. Apply matte white eyeshadow to the base of the lid, along the inner corner, and under the brow bone.

5. Apply dark brown eyeshadow along the top crease and softly along the lower lashline, making the shadow on the outer corner of the upper and lower lashline connect.

6. Curl lashes and apply black mascara to the upper and lower eyelashes.

7. Apply short and long individual eyelashes, alternately, to the outer corner of the eye.

8. Apply ash blond eyebrow powder.

9. Apply clear brow gel.

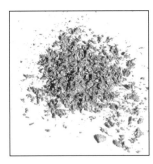

Classic

There is something regal about wearing red lipstick. It's timeless, feminine, and always glamorous. Pairing red lips with the wrong eye makeup can turn regal into trashy instantly. Red lips are paired best with neutral eyes. Use soft shimmers for added radiance.

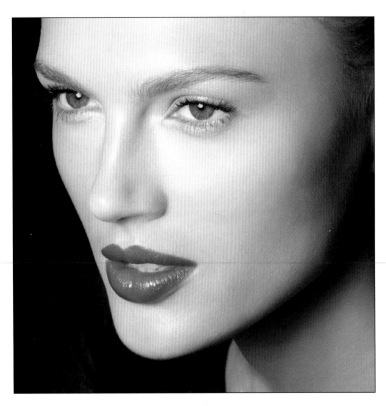

1. Apply beige foundation to the eyelid and undereye.

2. Apply beige stick concealer to the inner corner and undereye.

3. Set the foundation and concealer with translucent loose powder.

4. Apply opal eyeshadow to the base of the lid and along the lower lashline as well as the inner corner of the eye.

5. Curl lashes and apply black mascara to the upper and lower eyelashes.

6. Apply short and long individual eyelashes to the corner of the eye.

7. Apply ash blond eyebrow powder.

8. Apply clear brow gel.

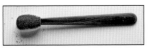

Sultry (Day to Night)

It's easy to take a daytime look and make it date night appropriate in just a few quick steps. Here the same eyeshadow colors are used to create the natural look on page 91, but a different application creates a smoldering eye.

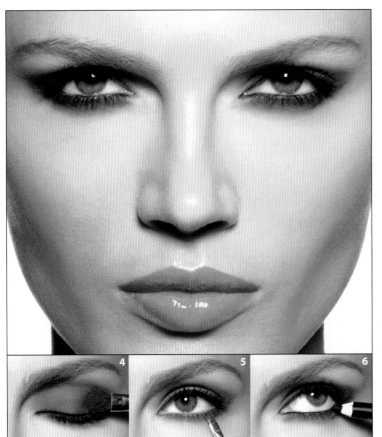

1. Apply beige foundation to the eyelid and undereye.

2. Apply beige stick concealer to the inner corner and undereye.

3. Set the foundation and concealer with translucent loose powder.

4. Apply dark brown eyeshadow to the base of the lid and on top of existing eyeshadow. This is the same brown that was used to contour the natural eye, only this time it is added to the base of the lid.

5. Smudge the same dark brown eyeshadow along the lower lashline.

6. Apply black pencil eyeliner inside the lower lashline.

7. Apply an extra coat of mascara to the existing mascara.

8. Apply a few long individual eyelashes on the outer corner.

9. Apply ash blond eyebrow powder.

10. Apply clear brow gel.

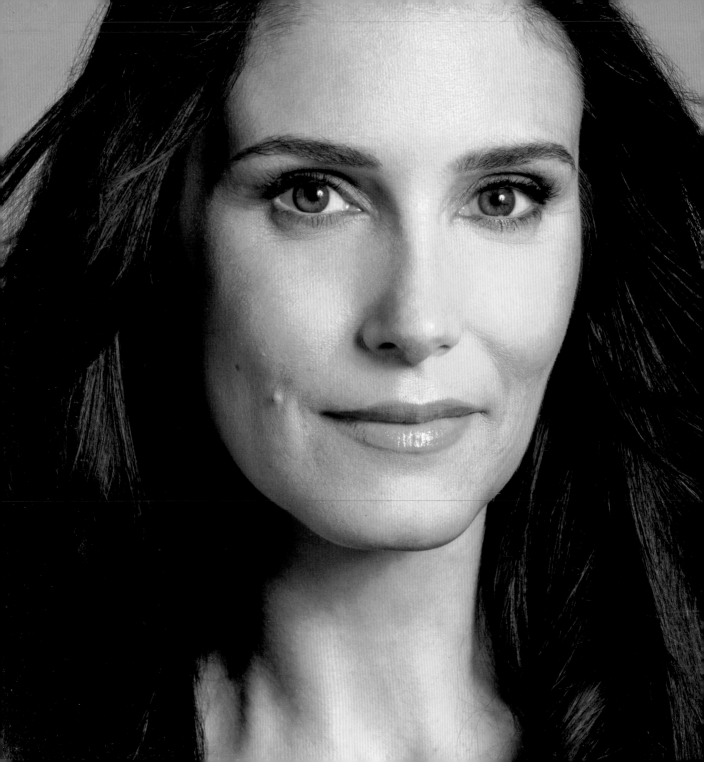

Eye Makeup at Every Age

I remember asking one of my seventysomething clients if it was okay to apply false eyelashes on her. She said she had never worn them before. (I don't know how she got through the sixties without them!) Needless to say, she loved them and has had me use them on her ever since. I think one of the biggest misconceptions about makeup is age-appropriate applications. Women often tell me, "I was told that because I'm over forty, I shouldn't wear shimmery eyeshadows." I find that absolutely ridiculous. Don't they know that forty is the new thirty?! A little shimmer on the eye is a great way to add a little youth to the eyes. I've also taught more over-fifty women than I can count how to apply a smoky eye. I truly believe that it's never too late to try new things. This chapter is all about changes you might experience around the eye area as you get older, and how to prevent as well as defy gravity. Never limit yourself and, remember, it's never too late to learn!

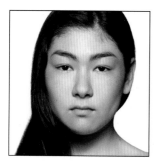

Teens

Less is more for teenagers—avoid clumpy mascara and black undereye shadow. Young skin often looks best with clean, natural-looking makeup. However, have fun with eye makeup as well—this is probably the only time in your life when you can wear glitter, crystals, and bright pink eyeshadow during the day and look fabulous. Experiment with color and try new looks. You're beautiful!

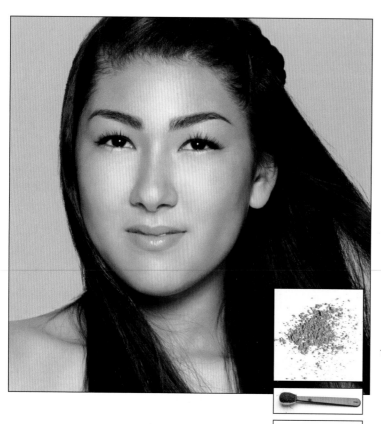

1. Apply warm beige foundation to the eyelid. (You can also use concealer or eyeshadow primer.)

2. Apply warm beige concealer to the inner corner of the eye.

3. Set the foundation and concealer with translucent loose powder.

4. Apply bright pink eyeshadow to the entire base of the lid.

5. Layer black eyeshadow along the upper lashline, slightly blending into the bright pink eyeshadow.

6. Apply white shimmering eyeshadow along the lower lashline.

7. Apply black cream eyeliner along the upper lashline and wing out corners slightly.

8. Curl lashes and apply volumizing mascara to the upper eyelashes.

9. Apply dark brown eyebrow pencil.

10. Apply clear brow gel.

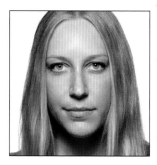

Twenties

The twenties are an important time for skin. Cell renewal starts to slow down. Thin skin around the eyes may start to develop fine lines. This is the time to start using a light eye cream with sunscreen that contains antioxidants to prevent cell damage. Avoid too much tugging of the eyes. Prevention is key to maintaining healthy skin, as well as developing routines to follow you into your thirties. Continue to have fun with makeup. Enjoy the perks of your twenties.

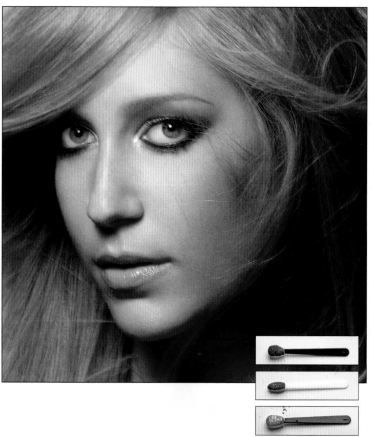

1. Apply beige foundation to the eyelid and undereye.

2. Apply light beige concealer to the inner corner and undereye.

3. Set the foundation and concealer with translucent loose powder.

4. Apply purple eyeshadow along the entire crease and outer corner, extending the shadow slightly.

5. Apply blue eyeshadow along the lower lashline and extend slightly outside the corner of the eye.

6. Apply black pencil eyeliner along the outer two-thirds of the upper lashline to bring the eye out.

7. Apply black pencil liner inside the lower rim of the eye and along the lower lashline, extending out.

8. Apply silver loose pigment shadow to the inside corner of the eye.

9. Curl lashes and apply black mascara to the upper and lower eyelashes.

10. Apply corner eyelashes on the corner of the eye.

11. Apply ash blond eyebrow powder.

12. Apply clear brow gel.

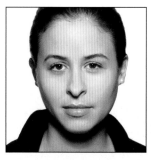

Thirties

If you haven't started your eye cream routine in your twenties, you're definitely going to want to start in your thirties. Fine lines become more visible as skin renewal becomes even slower. Light eye creams that also contain ingredients that encourage cellular turnover are crucial. Skin cells renew themselves at night, so an eye cream for night is especially important in your thirties and thereafter. I recommend ones that contain vitamin C and antioxidants.

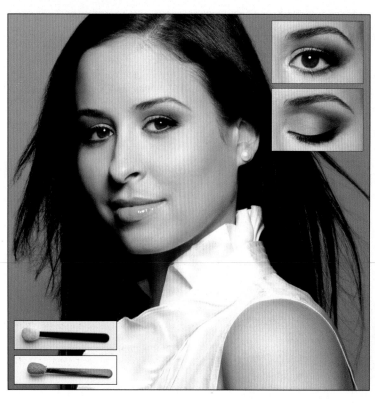

1. Apply warm beige foundation to the eyelid and undereye.

2. Apply beige concealer to the inner corner of the eye.

3. Set the foundation and concealer with translucent loose powder.

4. Apply shimmery pale rose eyeshadow to the base of the lid and along the inner corner.

5. Apply dark rose eyeshadow on the outer corner and along the outer third of the lower lashline, slightly extending the eyeshadow.

6. Apply dark purple eyeshadow along the upper and lower outer corners, slightly extending the eyeshadow.

7. Apply black cream eyeliner along the upper lashline, applying thicker at the ends to lift the eyes up and out.

8. Apply black cream eyeliner along the outer two-thirds of the lower lashline.

9. Curl lashes and apply black mascara to the upper and lower eyelashes.

10. Apply short and long individual eyelashes at the outer corner of the eye to add extra lift and extend the eye.

11. Apply soft brown eyebrow pencil, focusing on the tail of the brow.

12. Apply clear brow gel.

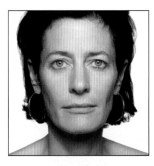

Forties Plus

I've met many women who never wore makeup until their forties or even fifties. They didn't see a need and didn't really care to learn until their eyes started to change. The eyelids and undereyes go through dramatic changes as you get older. Skin texture thins out and sagging begins on the upper and lower lids. Fine lines graduate into wrinkles. When looking for eye creams, which are essential at this point, look for products that promote cell renewal and rebuild collagen.

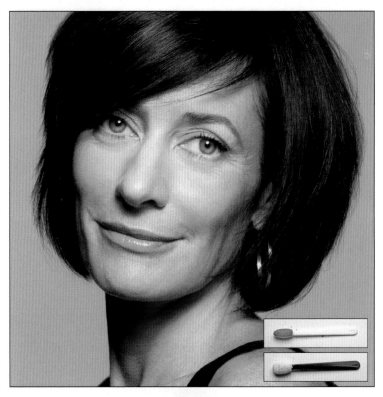

1. Apply warm beige foundation to the eyelid and undereye.

2. Apply creamy beige concealer to the inner corner and undereye.

3. Set the foundation and concealer with translucent loose powder.

4. Apply golden beige eyeshadow to the base of the lid.

5. Apply white eyeshadow under the brow bone to lightly accentuate eyebrow.

6. Apply a thick line of dark brown cream eyeliner to the outer corner of the upper lashline.

7. Apply light beige eyeliner to the inside rim of the lower lashline to cut out red and open up the eye.

8. Curl lashes and apply waterproof black mascara to the upper and lower eyelashes.

9. Apply corner eyelashes on the outer corner.

10. Apply medium brown eyebrow pencil, focusing on lifting the brows. (See page 103.)

Taylor's Tip

Use beige or off-white liner inside the lower rims of the eyes to cut redness and brighten. This opens up the eyes and makes them appear less fatigued.

Taylor's Tip

When applying eye makeup, focus on "lifting" the eyes. Add color to your eyeshadow routine. Avoid the habit of wearing eyeliner just along the lower lashline; it can make eyes appear saggy. Focus on the eyelids instead. Brown shades can look muddy, so choose golds and mauves as well as blue-grays, which look great on everyone.

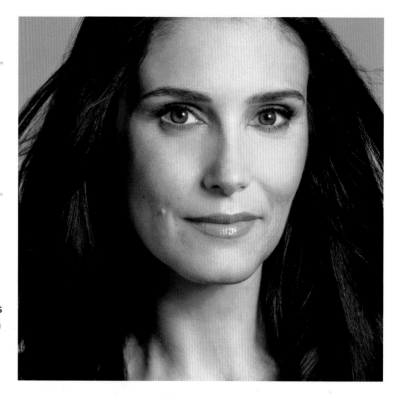

Simple Age-Defying Tips

I've met more than a few women while doing appearances throughout the country who have put all their energy into something or someone other than themselves, essentially deciding that it was no longer important to take care of themselves. Then the kids go off to college and they find themselves wondering when they stopped paying attention. Having kids myself that are only a few years away from going to college (When did that happen?), I must say that they take more pride in themselves when they have a good example to follow. And when you're confident and feel good about yourself, everyone around you is happier. Everyone has five minutes to spare to take care of themselves. While it may take a little longer than that the first few times around, the more you practice these makeup techniques, the faster you'll get.

The idea behind all this is to "bring the eye up." These techniques will camouflage and minimize droopiness in the lids, brows, lashes, and skin, making the eyes—and the whole face—instantly appear more youthful.

The Eye-Lifting Power of an Eyelash Curler

Curling lashes adds instant lift to the eyes. Droopy eyes look ten years younger with perky lashes. The newly standing lashes also push back drooping lids, adding renewed youth to the eyes. Use a prestige brand curler—it really does make a difference. Curl eyelashes for a few seconds each at the base, middle, and tip of the lashes before applying mascara to create an instant open, youthful eye. (See page 29.)

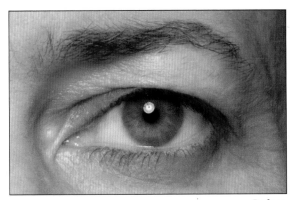
Before

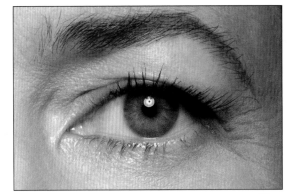
After

Minimize Crow's Feet Using Concealer

Fine lines and wrinkles create darkness in the outer corners of the eyes. The lines cast shadows, making fine lines even more apparent. Applying a concealer at an upward angle after all other makeup is on gives the illusion of lift to the eyes. Use a concealer brush and wipe across the corners at a 45-degree angle to clean up any eyeliner errors and erase fine lines. Use cream or pen concealers, as they are less likely to settle into fine lines.

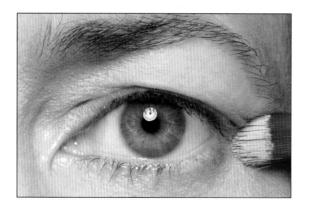

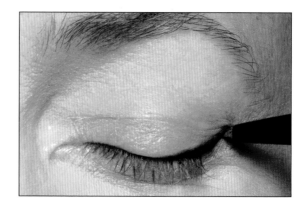

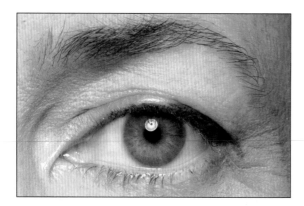

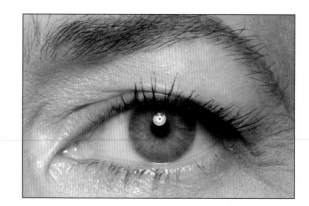

Taylor's Tip

For mature eyelids, use cream eyeliner to minimize pulling and movement.

Instant Eyelift with Eyeliner

Apply dark brown or black eyeliner on the upper outer corners of the eyes at a 45-degree angle to create the illusion of lift to the eye. Try cream eyeliners in a pot. Look for smudge-proof types. Cream eyeliners don't tug at the skin; use with a soft, small shadow detail brush for the best results.

Lift Brows Without Botox

As we age, the ends of our eyes and eyebrows start to sag. When filling or drawing in brows, don't follow the brow line. Instead, go above the brow line and use a brow gel to hold hairs up. As skin loses elasticity, the tails of the brows tend to fall. This draws the eyes down. Use pencil or pomade to add height to the tails of the brows. Tweeze underneath if necessary. This adds instant lift, creating a more youthful brow. Use a pale eyeshadow under the brow bone to accentuate the area.

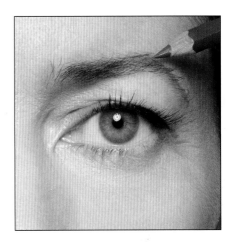

The brows also tend to thin with age, growing sparse and unruly. Cut away any excess and fill in brows using powder or a pencil. Look for brow colors that are one to two shades lighter than your hair color and in the same color family. For women with brows that are a different shade from their hair, look for a brow color in between the two to create flow. For example, if you have warm brown hair and black eyebrows, fill in your brows using a soft brown to help unify the hair and brows.

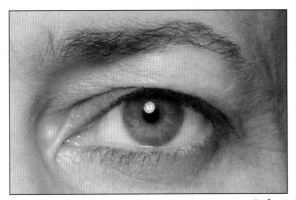

Before

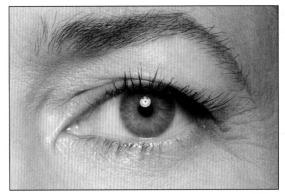

After

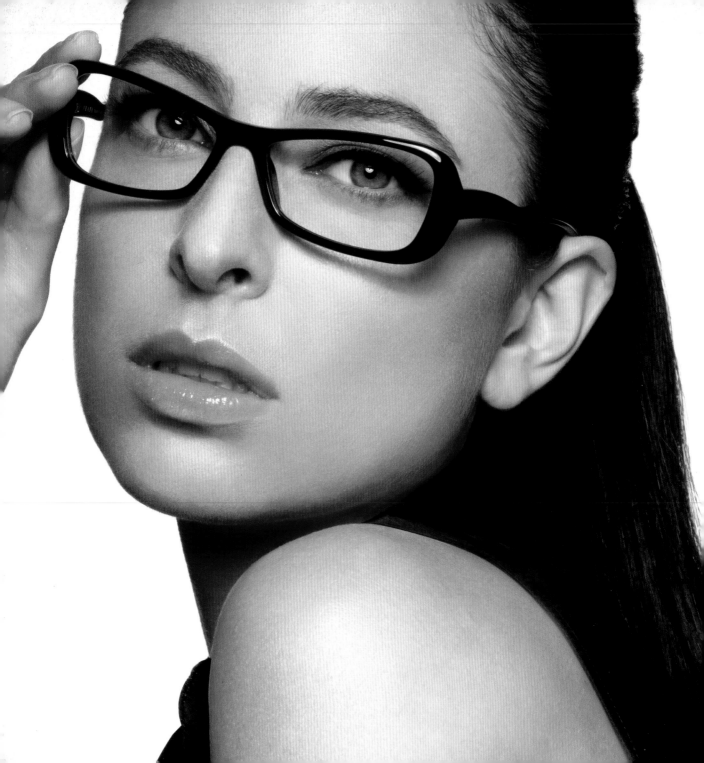

Eyeglasses: Standing Out from Behind the Lens

Eyeglasses are incredibly sexy. And a little makeup goes a long way. It doesn't take much to create gorgeous eyes. Many eyeglass wearers don't bother with eye makeup because they think it's pointless since their eyes are hidden behind frames, but that is even more reason to take extra care with the eyes, since the glasses make the eyes the focal point of the face.

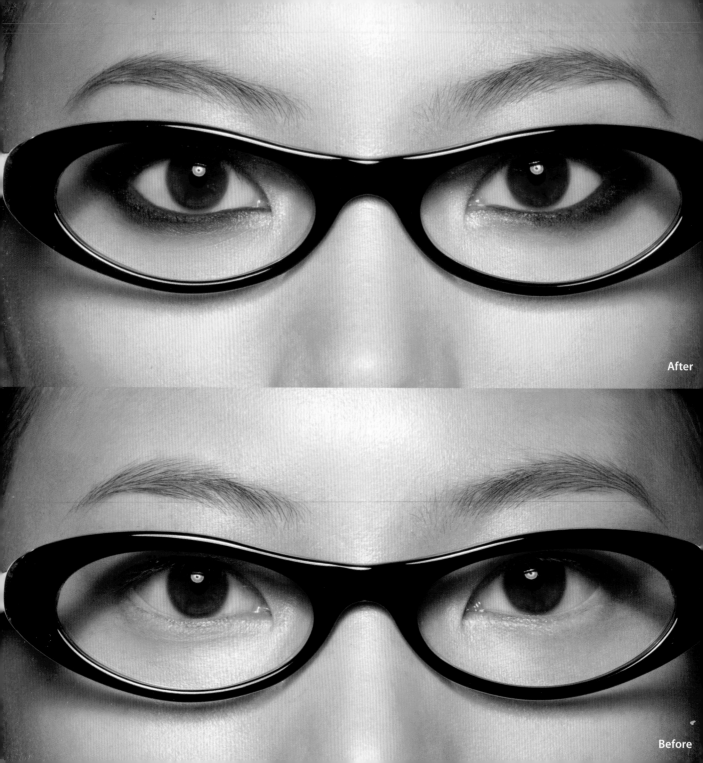

After

Before

Eyeglass Makeover—
Before and After

Here a little eye makeup and eyebrow pencil make simple eyes sultry in a few easy steps. It changes the look completely.

1. Apply warm beige foundation to the eyelid and undereye.
2. Apply stick beige concealer to the inner corner of the eye.
3. Set the foundation and concealer with translucent loose powder.
4. Apply waterproof black liner along the upper and lower lashlines, and inside the lower rim, slightly extending to bring the eye out.
5. Gently smudge black liner using black eyeshadow and an eyeshadow smudge brush.
6. Apply shimmery white eyeshadow to the inner corner.
7. Apply black cream eyeliner along the upper lashline.
8. Curl lashes and apply waterproof black mascara to the upper and lower eyelashes.
9. Apply dark brown eyebrow pomade using a synthetic angled brow brush, concentrating on slightly extending the tail of the brow.
10. Apply clear brow gel.

Taylor's Tip

What comes first: the eye makeup or the contacts? The answer is the contacts. It's too messy to try to put contacts in after eye-makeup application. Make sure to blink often so that your contacts don't dry out.

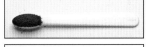

Frames

The type of frame that you wear says a lot about who you are. Are they frameless, simple and professional, no fuss, or are they bold and striking? Do they have a period look to them? It's important to find the best frames, since they are a daily part of every eyeglass wearer's look.

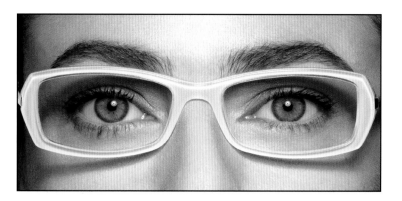

White Frames

White frames offer a clean linear look. When applying eyeshadow, try a wash that complements your eye color. Here a cool gray is a great option to bring out the eyes.

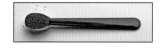

1. Apply beige foundation to the eyelid and undereye.

2. Apply light beige concealer to the inner corner of the eye.

3. Set the foundation and concealer with translucent loose powder.

4. Apply cool gray eyeshadow to the base of the lid and along the lower lashline.

5. Curl lashes and apply black mascara to the upper and lower eyelashes.

6. Apply dark ash brown eyebrow pencil.

7. Apply clear brow gel.

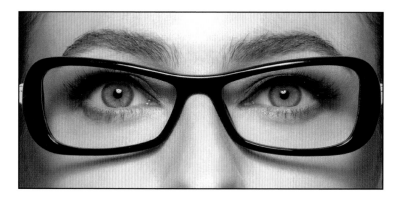

Large Black Frames

While black frames can look very cool, eyes can disappear behind them and the shape of the eyes can appear nonexistent. Use liner to define, and add some lashes to add femininity. If you find that your eyelashes hit your glasses, make sure to curl your eyelashes.

1. Apply beige foundation to the eyelid and undereye.
2. Apply light beige concealer to the inner corner of the eye.
3. Set the foundation and concealer with translucent loose powder.
4. Apply cool gray eyeshadow to the base of the lid and on the outer corner of the lower lashline.
5. Apply black cream eyeliner along the upper lashline.
6. Curl lashes and apply black mascara to the upper and lower eyelashes.
7. Apply short and long individual eyelashes to the outer corner of the eye.
8. Apply dark ash brown eyebrow pencil.
9. Apply clear brow gel.

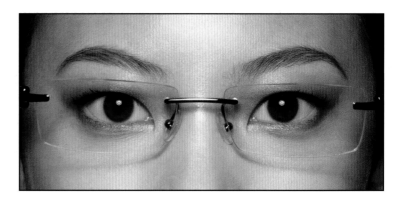

Clear Frames

When I see clear frames, I think of a person who is no-nonsense, a bit serious, and focused. It is especially important for clear-frame wearers to wear at least eyeliner for definition, or eyes can tend to look washed out. Try neutral shadow colors, simple and clean, that don't overpower.

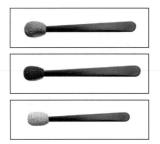

1. Apply warm beige foundation to the eyelid and undereye.
2. Apply stick beige concealer to the inner corner of the eye.
3. Set the foundation and concealer with translucent loose powder.
4. Apply soft warm copper eyeshadow to the base of the lid and along the lower lashline.
5. Apply dark warm brown eyeshadow to the lower base of the lid, blending into the copper shadow and along the lower outer corner, extending the eye out slightly.
6. Apply gold shimmer eyeshadow along the inner corner and under the brow bone.
7. Apply black cream eyeliner along the upper lashline.
8. Curl lashes and apply waterproof black mascara to the upper and lower eyelashes.
9. Apply dark brown eyebrow pomade, concentrating on the tail of the brow.
10. Apply clear brow gel.

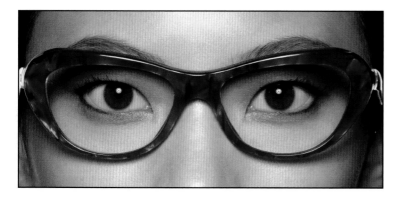

Colored Frames

Colored frames are fun ways of showing off your personality. When choosing eye makeup colors, it is important to look to the color of the frame for inspiration so that it all blends harmoniously. The colors don't need to be exact matches; in fact, they shouldn't be. Just keep them in the same color family. Here the lightest color of the frame, pale pink, guides the look.

1. Apply warm beige foundation to the eyelid and undereye.
2. Apply stick beige concealer to the inner corner of the eye.
3. Set the foundation and concealer with translucent loose powder.
4. Apply soft rose eyeshadow to the base of the lid and along the lower lashline.

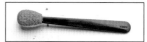
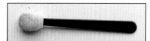

5. Apply pale pink shimmering eyeshadow in the inner corner and under the brow bone.
6. Apply black cream eyeliner along the upper and lower lashlines.
7. Curl lashes and apply waterproof black mascara to the upper and lower eyelashes.
8. Apply dark brown eyebrow pomade using a synthetic angled brow brush, concentrating on slightly extending the tail of the brow.
9. Apply clear brow gel.

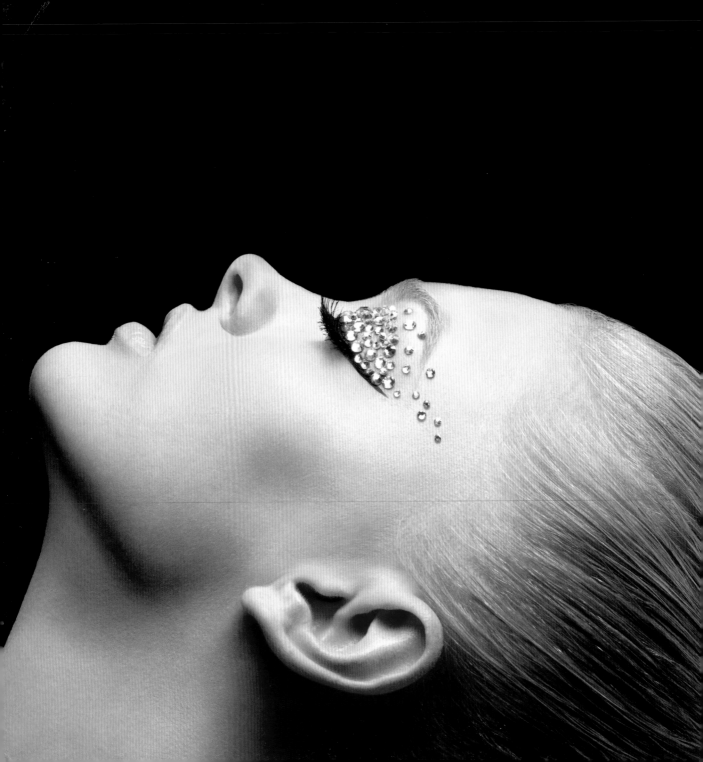

Inspirations and Eye-Cons

Inspirations

The beauty of the world inspires me. The history of beauty inspires me. I don't just look to the current runway trends to tell me what beautiful is. I look to nature, icons of the past, and the women I meet every day. The next time you look at a flower, a butterfly, or a painting, pay attention to the use of color and texture and how they intermix. You'll surely become inspired and moved to create a look of your own.

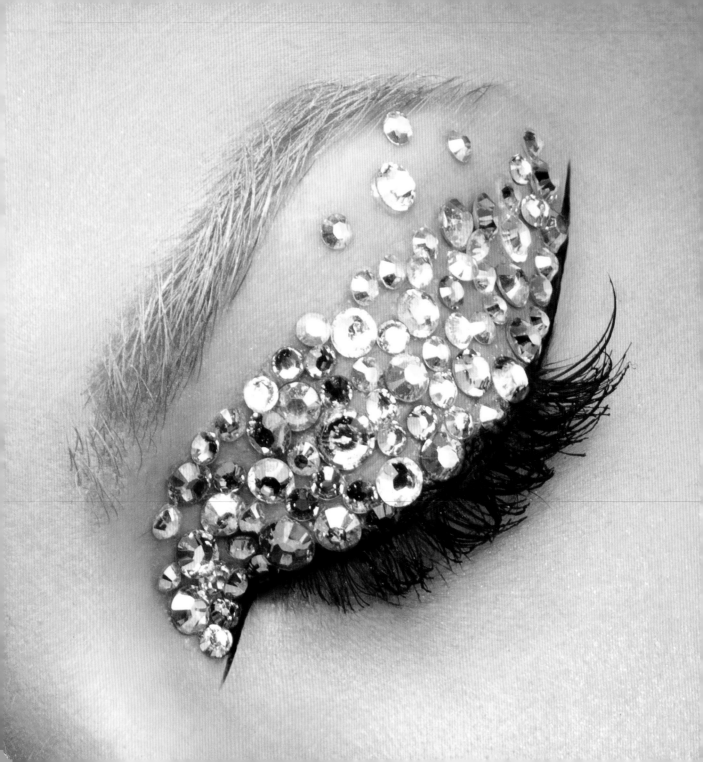

Crystals

Who says makeup has to be only about eyeshadow and eyeliner? High-end crystals make a statement and have been used for decades in the fashion, beauty, and music industries. Highly stylized ballerinas of the twenties often wore crystals on their lids and were considered some of the most beautiful women of their time. Use only a few for subtle fun or add several to create a jeweled eye.

Crystals in several different sizes and colors were used to create this look. White, crystalline, pink, and yellow-green crystals in various sizes were applied sporadically across the eyelid using eyelash glue and tweezers while the model was lying down with her eyes closed. To achieve the same effect at home:

1. Surgical eye glue adheres better to clean skin, so remove any makeup on the eyelid.

2. Apply ivory concealer to the inner corner and undereye.

3. Set concealer with translucent loose powder.

4. Curl lashes and apply volumizing mascara to the upper and lower lashes. Apply short lashes over the entire lid and long individual lashes at the outer corner. (It's more difficult to do this once the crystals are on.)

5. Apply white brow mascara and set with white eyeshadow.

6. Use flat head tweezers to hold the crystal, and dip the flat side of the stone in surgical eyelash adhesive (available at drugstores). Allow for it to get tacky (you can blow on it if necessary). With the head tilted back, apply white, crystalline, pink, yellow, and green crystals in various sizes sporadically across the lid, with a concentration of pink at the beginning of the lid and green at the end of the lid. Here I started at the inner corner along the lashline and worked my way up and out toward the brow and the outer corner of the eye.

7. Finish off with a thin line of black liquid liner at the base of the lid.

8. Allow the stones to dry on the lid before any activity.

Taylor's Tip

Avoid using extra-hold glue, which normally comes in clear form in a small glass bottle, as it can be difficult and painful to remove. Remove crystals gently using eye makeup remover made specifically for waterproof makeup.

Taylor's Tip

If you are attempting this look on yourself, do not lie down. Instead, tilt your head, look down, and apply the first row along the entire upper lashline. The crystals will slightly fall since you are upright, so give yourself a little bit of room. Work your way up in rows, allowing each row to dry completely before applying the next layer. Try applying the crystals only above or below your natural crease to avoid discomfort.

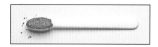

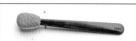

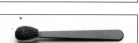

Flora

Flowers are an amazing source for color inspiration, as nature does it best. Flowers always seem to have the right blend of color, whether it's pale, soft, or vibrant. Here the colors from a hydrangea provide the palette, pulling the hint of vibrant blue from the center of the flower and using that for the inner corner of the eyes, then fading it into soft green and finally pink, duplicating the hydrangea leaves.

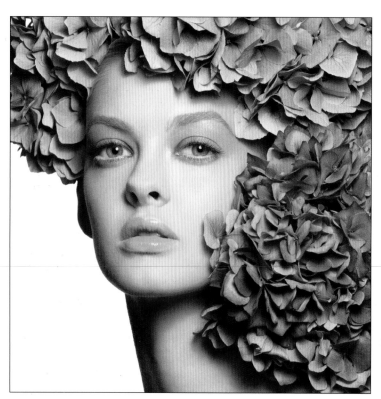

1. Apply pale beige foundation to the eyelid and undereye.

2. Apply ivory concealer to the inner corner of the eye.

3. Set the foundation and concealer with translucent loose powder.

4. Apply shimmering light green eyeshadow to the first two-thirds of the upper lid, starting at the inner corner.

5. Apply warm pink shadow to the final third of the upper lid.

6. Apply royal blue shadow in the inner corner of the eye.

7. Apply shimmering light green eyeshadow along the lower lashline.

8. Apply pale beige eyeliner to the inner rim of the eye.

9. Curl lashes and apply black mascara to the upper and lower eyelashes.

10. Apply long individual eyelashes sporadically across the upper eyelid.

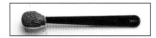

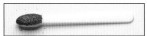

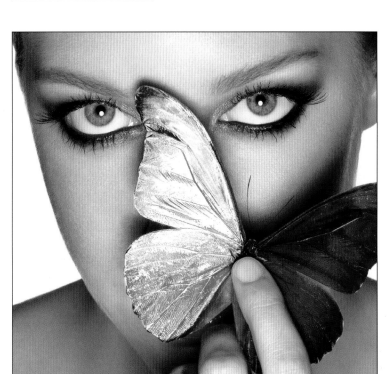

Fauna

Nature is full of beauty and inspiration, whether it's the colors of the sky, birds, or butterflies. Pulling colors from nature's creatures offers incredible ideas and color combinations.

1. Apply beige foundation to the eyelid and undereye.

2. Apply light beige concealer to the inner corner and undereye.

3. Set the foundation and concealer with translucent loose powder.

4. Apply purple eyeshadow along the entire crease and outer corner, extending the shadow slightly.

5. Apply blue eyeshadow along the lower lashline and extend slightly beyond the outer corner of the eye.

6. Apply black pencil eyeliner along two-thirds of the upper lashline to bring the eye out.

7. Apply black pencil eyeliner inside the lower rim of the eye and along the lower lashline, extending out.

8. Apply white loose pigment shadow to the inside corner of the eye.

9. Curl lashes and apply black mascara to the upper and lower eyelashes.

10. Apply corner eyelashes on the corner of the eye.

11. Apply ash blond eyebrow powder.

12. Apply clear brow gel.

When applying eyeshadow, shake off the excess and tap it on—as opposed to using a side-to-side motion—to minimize fallen eyeshadow. To make cleanup easier, apply eye makeup before the rest of your makeup.

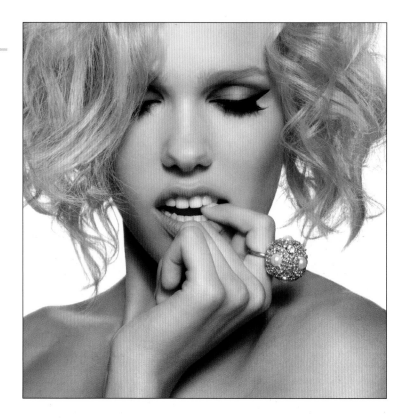

Eye-Cons

Throughout the decades (and even the centuries), eye makeup has played a large role in the classic looks of the period. Think of the iconic eyeliner look of the fifties. And after all, what would Twiggy have been without her lashes? Each decade offers a new take on eye makeup, and it inspires the looks of today—and the future.

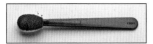

The Vamp

Inspired by the ultimate vamp of the 1920s, Theda Bara, who often played the sultry femme fatale on the silent screen, this look remains a classic for women of all ages.

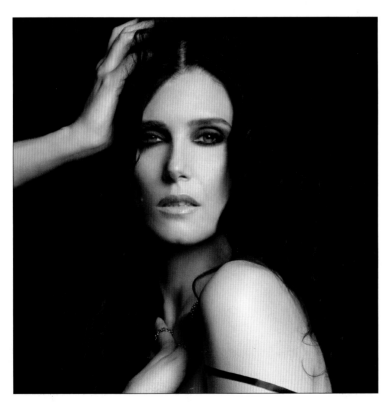

1. Apply light beige foundation to the eyelid and undereye.

2. Apply ivory concealer to the inner corner of the eye.

3. Set the foundation and concealer with translucent loose powder.

4. Apply black eyeshadow along the entire base of the lid slightly above the crease, wrapping the color around the entire eye, including the lower lashline.

5. Apply black cream eyeliner along the upper lashline.

6. Apply black pencil eyeliner inside the lower rim of the eye.

7. Curl lashes and apply black mascara to the upper and lower eyelashes.

8. Apply short and long individual eyelashes on the outer corner of the eye.

9. Apply brown eyebrow pencil, concentrating on the tail of the brow.

The Original Diva

Amy Winehouse wasn't the first to popularize strong, lifted eyeliner. The legendary opera singer Maria Callas wasn't considered classically beautiful when she was younger, so she created her own look and made herself an iconic beauty.

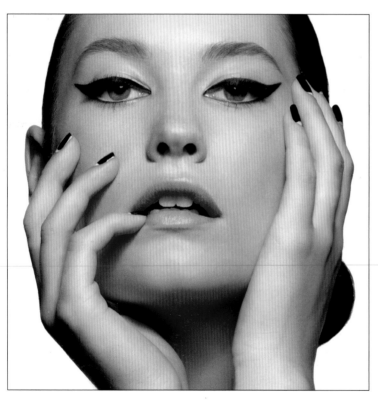

1. Apply light beige foundation to the eyelid and undereye.

2. Apply ivory concealer to the inner corner of the eye.

3. Set the foundation and concealer with translucent loose powder.

4. Apply a thick line of black cream eyeliner to the upper lashline, winging the ends up at an 80-degree angle, almost perpendicular to the eye.

5. Apply a thin line of black cream eyeliner to the lower lashline.

6. Curl lashes and apply lengthening black mascara to the upper and lower eyelashes.

7. Apply a short eyelash strip along the upper lashline.

8. Apply light beige eyeliner inside the lower rim of the eye.

9. Apply dark medium brown eyebrow pencil, concentrating on a sharp tail to each brow.

10. Apply clear brow gel.

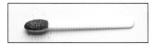

Living Doll

Before the fifties, most dolls represented children. The advent of Barbie and other "fashion dolls" led to dolls whose clothes, hair, and makeup displayed a grown-up look. Pale blue eyeshadow, thick liner on the upper lid, and great lashes were staples in most women's boudoirs during this time.

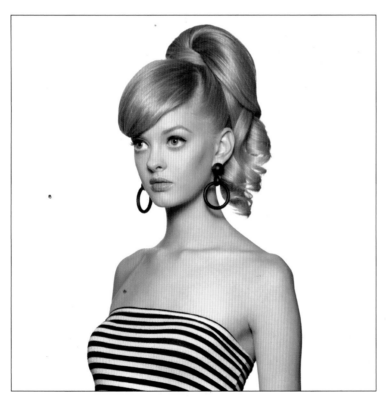

1. Apply pale beige foundation to the eyelid and undereye.

2. Apply ivory concealer to the inner corner of the eye.

3. Set the foundation and concealer with translucent loose powder.

4. Apply pale blue eyeshadow along the base of the lid.

5. Apply black cream eyeliner in medium thickness along the upper lashline.

6. Apply pale beige cream eyeliner inside the lower rim of the eye.

7. Curl lashes and apply volumizing black mascara to the upper and lower eyelashes.

8. Apply long individual eyelashes along the center of the lid.

9. Apply medium ash eyebrow powder.

10. Apply clear brow gel.

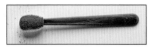

Gamine

Penelope Tree was a late sixties model who was famous for her exotic, almost alien, look and her long legs and even longer lashes. She made such a strong impact during her time that "the Tree" will forever be remembered as an emblem of the swinging sixties and an icon of beauty and fashion.

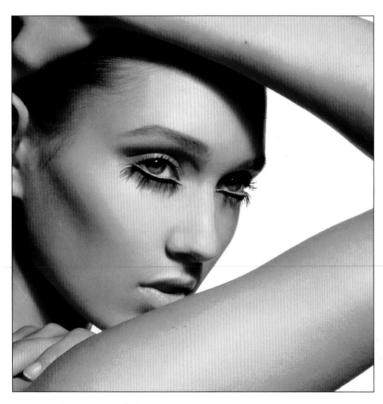

1. Apply warm beige foundation to the eyelid and undereye.

2. Apply beige concealer to the inner corner of the eye.

3. Set the foundation and concealer with translucent loose powder.

4. Apply white eyeshadow to the base of the lid.

5. Apply dark brown eyeshadow along the crease.

6. Apply dark brown eyeshadow along the lower lashline.

7. Apply black cream eyeliner along the lower lashline.

8. Apply white pencil eyeliner in the lower rim of the eye.

9. Curl lashes and apply black mascara to the upper and lower eyelashes.

10. Apply chunks of long individual eyelashes along the lower lashline.

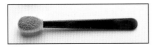
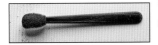

Disco Diva

What would the seventies be without Diana Ross? Her makeup looks were a signature of the decade. Sporadic lash application and glossy lids reign supreme for this look.

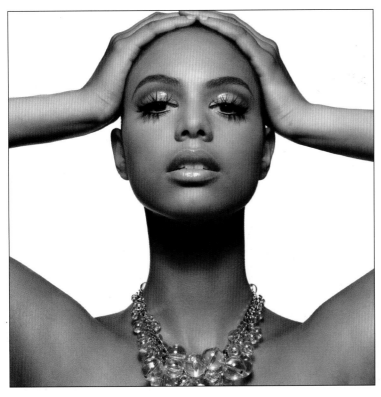

1. Apply honey foundation to the eyelid and undereye.

2. Apply light golden concealer to the inner corner of the eye.

3. Set the foundation and concealer with orange loose powder.

4. Apply taupe eyeshadow to the base of the lid and brow bone.

5. Apply warm brown eyeshadow to the outer corner to add lift to the eye.

6. Apply black cream eyeliner along the upper lashline and lower outer corner.

7. Apply white eyeliner in the lower rim of the eye.

8. Curl lashes and apply full-volume black mascara to the upper and lower eyelashes.

9. Apply chunks of long individual lashes sporadically along the upper lashline. This can also be achieved by cutting a full strip into several pieces.

10. Apply dark brown eyebrow powder.

11. Apply clear brow gel.

12. Apply clear eyegloss over the entire lid.

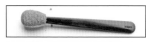
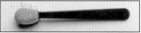
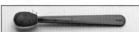

New Romantic

When I was growing up in the eighties, one of my first experiences with makeup occurred in a convenience store. I couldn't take my eyes off a magazine cover featuring a man wearing simply stunning eye makeup. Here's one of the iconic looks of that time.

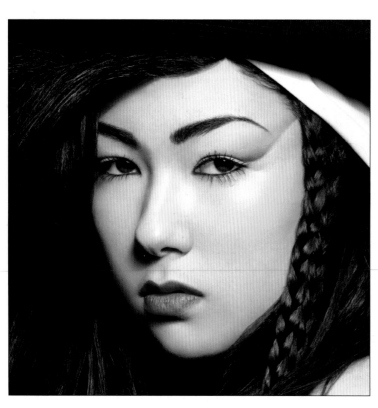

1. Apply light beige foundation to the eyelid and undereye.

2. Apply light beige concealer to the inner corner of the eye.

3. Set the foundation and concealer with translucent loose powder.

4. Apply rust-colored eyeshadow from the top of the upper outer crease and create a sharp angled line to the temple.

5. Apply yellow eyeshadow on the remaining upper lid, remaining above the crease to the brow bone.

6. Apply black eyeshadow under the rust, creating a lifted line.

7. Apply white eyeshadow under the black and rust shadow, drawing out to the temple.

8. Apply black pencil eyeliner inside the lower rim of the eye.

9. Curl lashes and apply black mascara to the upper and lower eyelashes.

10. Apply dark brown eyebrow pomade to the brow, creating a heavy dark eyebrow.

11. Apply clear brow gel.

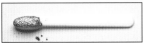

The Future

We've seen the different makeup looks of the past. And I'm more than curious to know what the future holds for us. Create your own futuristic look based on what suits your eye shape and attitude.

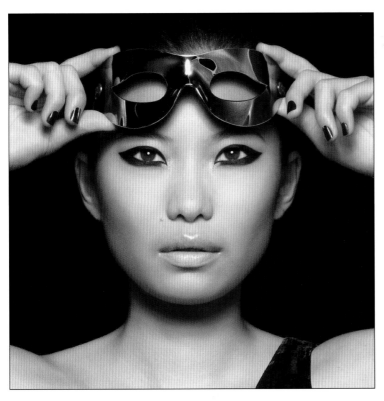

1. Apply warm beige foundation to the eyelid and undereye.

2. Apply beige concealer under the inner corner of the eye.

3. Set the foundation with translucent loose powder.

4. Apply black cream eyeliner along the upper and lower lashlines, creating a shape similar to a leaf.

5. Apply black waterproof eyeliner to the lower inner rim of the eye.

6. Apply silver shimmer to the inner corner.

7. Curl lashes and apply waterproof black mascara to the upper and lower eyelashes.

8. Apply warm brown eyebrow pomade.

9. Apply clear brow gel.

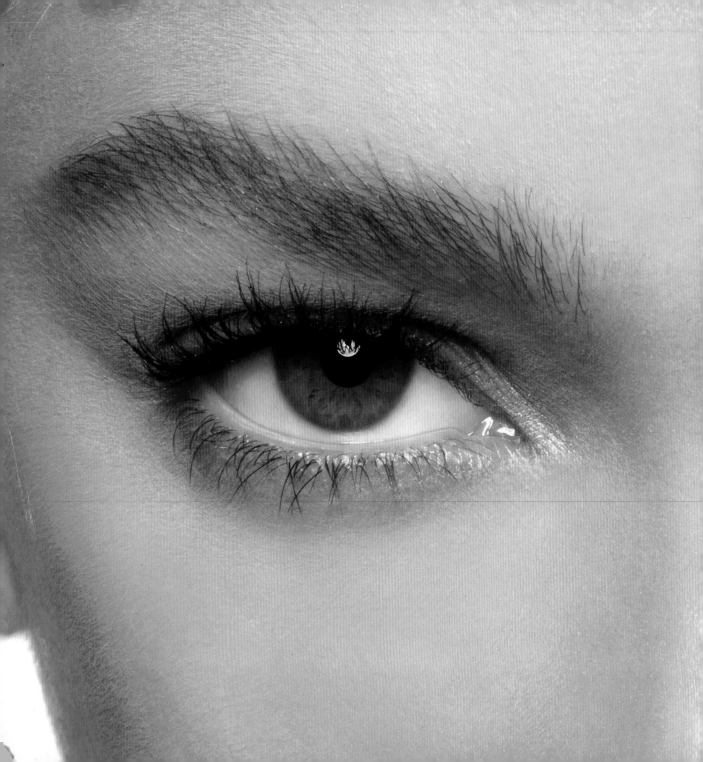

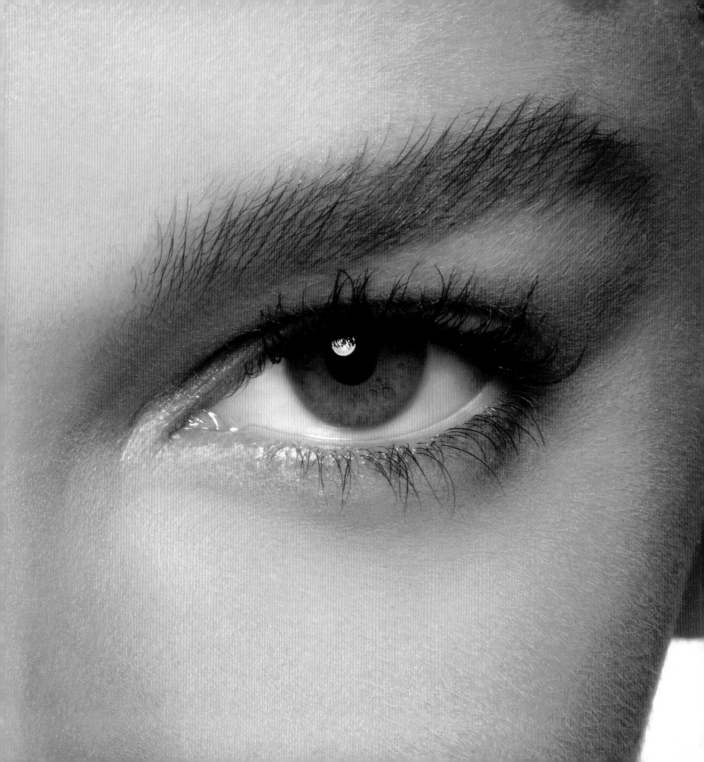

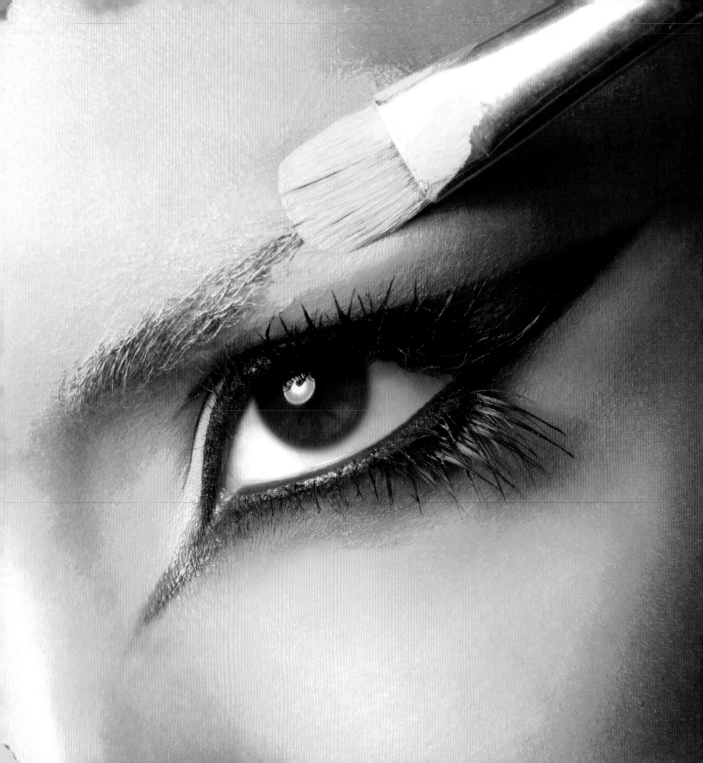

Acknowledgments

Heartfelt Gratitude

First and foremost, I would like to thank God for all of his blessings. I am grateful for the past, good and bad, which has made me who I am today.

All my love and thanks to my husband, Raffi, and beautiful teenagers, Adina and Christopher. You guys make everything easier and add laughter and joy to my life. Thank you for always being there for me and supporting all my sometimes nutty endeavors. Thank you for being the assistants, models, cleaning crew, and craft services, and the best family anyone can ask for. I love you more than words.

My undying gratitude goes to those of you who gave of your time and held me up when I was down and needed support the most. You went above and beyond what you needed to, selflessly, and made this book your own. To Albert Sanchez, you are a *genius* photographer in all ways, and your talent and amazing attitude made this book what it is. To Pedro Zalba, you've helped me grow as an artist with your creative direction and fantastic energy. Thank you for putting all of yourself into this project. I am truly blessed to have both of you in my life. Your infinite knowledge of beauty and fashion took this book to the next level and inspires me.

To Kita Huynh, thank you for multitasking during this tough time; it was very much needed and appreciated. Manuel Benevides, thank you for all your help and being there for me, even when it was last-minute.

It truly meant a lot. To Jason Stanton and Paul Anthony Castro, thank you for your talents and late nights. I will always remember the love and support you showed me. To John Shin and Rondi Ballard, thank you for being part of another great project and giving of your time and talent.

Thank you to everyone at Perigee. Jeanette Shaw, thank you so much for your support, kindness, and infinite patience. To Tiffany Estreicher, thank you so much for your efforts and for putting so much into this project. Thank you to John Duff, my publisher, for another incredible opportunity.

To Melissa Flashman, my wonderful literary agent, and everyone at Trident Media Group: Thank you for being such an incredible support system. Educating women to find their own beauty is my passion, and all of you help make it possible.

To everyone at the Cloutier Remix. I'm grateful to be a part of the best. Madeline Leonard, you have helped me grow so much. You have nurtured every part of my career, and your excitement always gives me renewed strength. Chantal Cloutier, thank you for all the support and kindness you've shown me. To Adrienne Novak, Susanna Burke, Brooke Bryant, Natalie Miller and Libby Anderson, Amy Sabel, Dequita Pettiford, Tanja Caldwell, and everyone at Cloutier past, present, and future: Your day-to-day efforts are what make my career—which is directly attached to my heart—go around.

Thank you to everyone at Luxottica and Lens Crafters for use of your amazing eyeglasses. To my friends Jadzia Tirsch, Nicole Cardillo, and Yee-Lynn, thank you for your wonderful support.

Thank you to all the models—professional and "real women"—for giving your time and lending me your beautiful faces: Shazia Ali, Mariah Bonner, Lisa Butler, Diana Chavez, Leza Cruz, Whitney Fransway, Alla Garkusha, April Geary, Caitlin Harroun, Kim Howe, Rachel Lehnen, Madeline Leonard, Danielle Lundquist, Lyndsay Magellan, Paula Miranda, Rina Sukhorukova, Joline Towers, and Julie Wolf. To the agents who make it all happen, I am truly grateful: Keith Carhill at Click Models, Jennifer Powell at Next Model Management, Victor Del Toro at Vision L.A., Luc Brinker at Wilhelmina, and Phira Luon at Photogenics.

Contributors

Albert Sanchez's first foray into image making was studying photo-realist painting in college. He was concurrently experimenting with photography, taking pictures of his glam rock friends and Barbie Dolls in phantasmagorical scenarios. His career in photography began in earnest in Paris as a portrait photographer and has since expanded into the fields of celebrity portraiture, fashion, and beauty. His notable subjects have included Nicole Kidman, Mick Jagger, and Dita Von Teese. He has shot beauty campaigns for MAC, Revlon, L'Oreal, and Tarina Tarantino Beauty. Drawing on his initial training in airbrushing, Albert enjoys being hands-on in the postproduction of his photography and is responsible for most of the image editing in this book.

Pedro Zalba first began participating on photo shoots as a set designer and prop stylist, working for top photographers such as Herb Ritts and Helmut Newton. For the last decade, he has worked exclusively with Albert Sanchez, collaborating on every aspect of image making, from conception through completion. Pedro would like to thank all the women who participated in this book: their beauty, in all its forms, colors, and ages, is an indefatigable source of inspiration.

Product photography by John Shin.

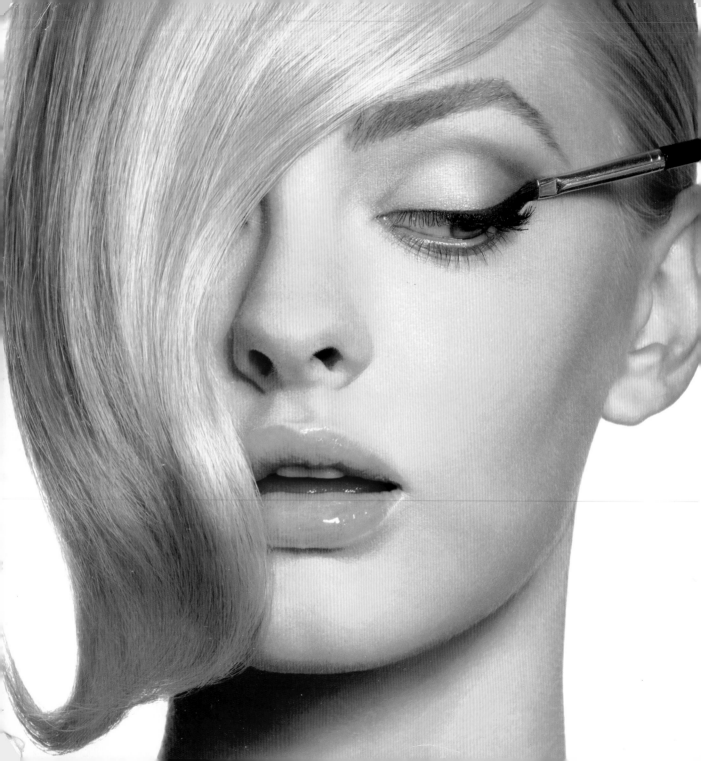